Dr. M. Penkman

# The Washington Manual™ Obstetrics and Gynecology Survival Guide

Faculty Advisors

**D. Michael Nelson, M.D., Ph.D.**
Virginia S. Lang Professor
Division of Maternal-Fetal Medicine
Washington University School of Medicine
St. Louis, Missouri

**Yoel Sadovsky, M.D.**
Associate Professor
Division of Maternal-Fetal Medicine
Washington University School of Medicine
St. Louis, Missouri

**Matthew A. Powell, M.D.**
Assistant Professor
Division of Gynecologic Oncology
Washington University School of Medicine
St. Louis, Missouri

**Neil S. Horowitz, M.D.**
Assistant Professor
Division of Gynecologic Oncology
Massachusetts General Hospital
Boston, Massachusetts

**Daniel B. Williams, M.D.**
Associate Professor
University of Cincinnati College of Medicine
Cincinnati, Ohio

**Anil B. Pinto, M.D., M.R.C.O.G., M.F.F.P.**
Private Practice
Baylor University Medical Center
Clinical Assistant Professor
University of Texas Southwestern Medical Center
Dallas, Texas

# The Washington Manual™ Obstetrics and Gynecology Survival Guide

Editors

## Jason Wright, M.D.
Division of Gynecologic Oncology
Department of Obstetrics and Gynecology
Washington University School of Medicine
St. Louis, Missouri

## Solange Wyatt, M.D.
Division of Maternal-Fetal Medicine
Department of Obstetrics and Gynecology
Washington University School of Medicine
St. Louis, Missouri

Series Editor

## Tammy L. Lin, M.D.
Adjunct Assistant Professor of Medicine
Washington University School of Medicine
St. Louis, Missouri

Series Advisor

## Daniel M. Goodenberger, M.D.
Professor of Medicine
Chief, Division of Medical Education
Washington University School of Medicine
Director, Internal Medicine Residency Program
Barnes-Jewish Hospital
St. Louis, Missouri

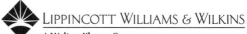
LIPPINCOTT WILLIAMS & WILKINS
A **Wolters Kluwer** Company
Philadelphia · Baltimore · New York · London
Buenos Aires · Hong Kong · Sydney · Tokyo

*Acquisitions Editors*: Danette Knopp and James Ryan
*Developmental Editors*: Scott Marinaro and Keith Donnellan
*Supervising Editor*: Mary Ann McLaughlin
*Production Editor*: Lucinda Ewing, Silverchair Science + Communications
*Manufacturing Manager*: Colin Warnock
*Cover Designer*: QT Design
*Compositor*: Silverchair Science + Communications
*Printer*: Victor Graphics

**©2003 by Department of Medicine, Washington University School of Medicine**

**Library of Congress Cataloging-in-Publication Data**
The Washington manual obstetrics and gynecology survival guide / [edited by] Jason Wright,
  Solange Wyatt.
    p. ; cm. -- (The Washington manual survival guide series)
  Includes bibliographical references and index.
  ISBN 0-7817-4363-X
   1. Pregnancy--Complications--Handbooks, manuals, etc. 2. Pregnancy--Handbooks, manuals, etc. 3. Prenatal care--Handbooks, manuals, etc. 4. Obstetrics--Handbooks, manuals, etc. 5. Gynecology--Handbooks, manuals, etc. I. Title: Manual obstetrics and gynecology survival guide. II. Wright, Jason. III. Wyatt, Solange. IV. Series.
   [DNLM: 1. Genital Diseases, Female--Handbooks. 2. Pregnancy Complications--Handbooks. 3. Prenatal Care--Handbooks. WQ 39 W319 2003]
RG571.W365 2003
618--dc21
                                                                                  2003047533

10 9 8 7 6 5 4 3 2 1

# Contents

# CONTENTS

# Chairman's Note

Medical knowledge is increasing at an exponential rate, and physicians are being bombarded with new facts at a pace that many find overwhelming. The Washington Manual™ Survival Guides were developed in this context for interns, residents, medical students, and other practitioners in need of readily accessible practical clinical information. They therefore meet an important need in an era of information overload.

I would like to acknowledge the authors who have contributed to these books. In particular, Tammy L. Lin, M.D., Series Editor, provided energetic and inspired leadership, and Daniel M. Goodenberger, M.D., Series Advisor, Chief of the Division of Medical Education in the Department of Medicine at Washington University, is a continual source of sage advice. The efforts and outstanding skill of the lead authors are evident in the quality of the final product. I am confident that this series will meet its desired goal of providing practical knowledge that can be directly applied to improving patient care.

Kenneth S. Polonsky, M.D.
Adolphus Busch Professor
Chairman, Department of Medicine
Washington University School of Medicine

# Series Preface

The Washington Manual™ Survival Guides, a multispecialty series, is designed to provide interns, residents, medical students, or anyone on the front lines of clinical care with quick, practical, essential information in an accessible format. It lets you hit the ground running as you learn the basics of practicing clinical medicine, gain more responsibility, and become a valued team member. Although written individually, they all incorporate series features. Each book takes care to give you an insider's view of how to get things done efficiently and effectively, tips on how to "survive" training, and pearls you will want to pass on in the future. It is similar to receiving a great sign-out from your favorite resident. When faced with an unfamiliar situation, we envision getting timely information and guidance from the survival guide (like you would from your resident) to make appropriate decisions at 3:00 p.m. or 3:00 a.m.

One of the most unique and notable features of this new series is that it was truly a joint effort across subspecialties at Washington University. We were fortunate to have significant departmental support, particularly from Kenneth Polonsky, M.D., whose commitment made this series possible. Every survival guide has the credibility of being written by recent interns, residents, or chief residents in that specialty with input from faculty advisors. We were fortunate to have found outstanding head authors who were not only highly regarded clinicians and teachers, but who also provided significant leadership and collaborated well together. Their incredible enthusiasm and desire to pass on their hard-earned knowledge, experiences, and wisdom clearly shine through in the series.

Anyone who has been through training will tell you the hours are long, the work is hard, and your energy is limited. With either a print or electronic version of a survival guide by your side, we hope you will work more efficiently, make decisions with more confidence, stay out of trouble, and get that ever-elusive good night's rest.

Tammy L. Lin, M.D., Series Editor
Daniel M. Goodenberger, M.D., Series Advisor

# Preface

Welcome to the first edition of *The Washington Manual™ Obstetrics and Gynecology Survival Guide*, a pocket manual that covers all the essential problems encountered in obstetrics and gynecology (OB/GYN). The manual was written by OB/GYN residents and fellows and encompasses the expertise of subspecialists in every field of OB/GYN. Our goal is to provide a succinct pocket manual that is a reference for the practice of OB/GYN.

All of the major fields of OB/GYN, including maternal-fetal medicine, reproductive endocrinology and infertility, gynecologic oncology, urogynecology, contraception, gynecologic infectious diseases, and general gynecology, are covered. Each of the major sections is divided into chapters, which in turn focus on a specific problem. The individual chapters contain diagnostic algorithms, tables of differential diagnosis, and management suggestions. Throughout the book, clinical pearls and common test questions are highlighted.

*The Washington Manual™ Obstetrics and Gynecology Survival Guide* provides practical information in an organized format and is essential for anyone involved in the practice of OB/GYN, family practice, internal medicine, pediatrics, or emergency medicine. OB/GYN is a fast-paced profession that is demanding but extremely rewarding. We wish you the best of luck in your OB/GYN clerkship, residency, or practice and hope that our manual is helpful in providing care to your patients.

We would like to thank D. Michael Nelson, M.D., Ph.D., Yoel Sadovsky, M.D., Matthew A. Powell, M.D., Neil S. Horowitz, M.D., Daniel B. Williams, M.D., and Anil B. Pinto, M.D., M.R.C.O.G., M.F.F.P., for serving as faculty advisors on this book.

J.D.W
S.M.W

# Key to Abbreviations

| | |
|---|---|
| AFI | amniotic fluid index |
| CVS | chorionic villus sampling |
| DHA | dehydroepiandrosterone |
| DHAS | dehydroepiandrosterone sulfate |
| DM | diabetes mellitus |
| DVP | deepest vertical pocket |
| EFM | external fetal monitor |
| fFN | fetal fibronectin |
| FLM | fetal lung maturity |
| FSE | fetal scalp electrode |
| GBBS | group B streptococcus |
| GCT | glucose challenge test |
| GFR | glomerular filtration rate |
| GTT | glucose tolerance test |
| HC/AC | head-to-abdominal circumference ratio |
| IUGR | intrauterine growth retardation |
| IUPC | intrauterine pressure catheter |
| IUPs | intrauterine pregnancies |
| LMP | low malignant potential |
| MSD | mean sac diameter |
| N/V | nausea and vomiting |
| NTDs | neural tube defects |
| OCPs | oral contraceptive pills |
| OD | ocular density |
| PACs | premature atrial contractions |
| PAPP-A | pregnancy-associated plasma protein A |
| PCOS | polycystic ovarian syndrome |
| PROM | premature rupture of membranes |
| PTL | preterm labor |
| PTU | propylthiouracil |
| PUBS | percutaneous umbilical blood sampling |
| SHBG | sex hormone–binding globulin |
| SSKI | supersaturated potassium iodide |
| TAS | transabdominal ultrasound |
| TVS | transvaginal ultrasound |

# Part One
# Obstetrics

# Keys to Survival

*Tips for success on obstetrics clerkship*

## THIRD YEAR CLINICAL CLERKSHIP

On the first day:

- Don't get overwhelmed.
- Follow junior residents and ask for instructions on which patients to see.
- Don't perform cervical exams without a resident.
- Follow all laboring patients.
- Introduce yourself to the nurses taking care of patients you are following.

## LABOR AND DELIVERY

- Be respectful of nurses; they'll teach you a lot.
- Labor notes:
  - Frequently review monitor strips for variability, accelerations, decelerations.
  - Cervical exams q2h.
  - Document progress of labor (Friedman curve).
- Keep senior residents updated on patients.
- Meds
  - Stress dose steroids if needed
  - Insulin for diabetics
- OB emergencies (call your senior resident for help)
  - Cord prolapse
  - Amniotic fluid embolism
  - Placental abruption
  - Precipitous delivery of multiples/breech
  - New-onset severe preeclampsia
  - Eclampsia

- Prolonged fetal deceleration
- Uterine rupture
- Maintain good communication with anesthesia.

## OBSTETRICS TRIAGE

- Don't get overwhelmed.
- Review dating criteria on all patients.
- Review vital signs on all patients.
  - BP, urine dip for protein
- Review previous c-section operative note on all vaginal birth after c-section candidates.
- Document fetal well-being.
  - Reactive nonstress test or biophysical profile
- Urgent evaluation required:
  - Vaginal bleeding
  - Preterm labor
- Don't be afraid to ask senior residents if you have questions.
- Don't perform digital exam in preterm patients with suspected premature rupture of membranes (PROM) until rupture of membranes ruled out.

# Antepartum Care

# 2 Physiologic Changes in Pregnancy

*A variety of physiologic changes occur during pregnancy*

## PHYSIOLOGIC CHANGES

Table 2-1 describes the physiologic changes that occur in pregnancy.

### TABLE 2-1.
### PHYSIOLOGIC CHANGES OF PREGNANCY

| | |
|---|---|
| Cardiovascular | |
| Cardiac output | Increased (43%) |
| Heart rate | Increased (17%) |
| Systemic vascular resistance | Decreased (21%) |
| Pulmonary vascular resistance | Decreased (34%) |
| Stroke volume | Increased (27%) |
| Systolic murmurs, split $S_1$ | |
| BP | Decreased (nadir second trimester) |
| Hematologic | |
| Blood volume | Increased (40–45%) |
| Hgb | Decreased (mean, 12.5 g/dL at term) |
| Fibrinogen | Increased (300–600 mg/dL) |
| Factor VII, VIII, IX, X | Increased |
| Factor XI, XIII | Decreased |
| PTT, PT | Decreased (very mild) |
| Antithrombin III, protein C | Unchanged |
| Protein S | Decreased |
| Plasminogen | Increased |
| Pulmonary | |
| Respiratory rate | Unchanged |
| Tidal volume | Increased (39%) |
| Minute ventilation | Increased (42%) |
| Functional residual capacity | Decreased (20%) |

*(continued)*

**TABLE 2-1.**
**(CONTINUED)**

| | |
|---|---|
| Residual volume | Decreased (20%) |
| Respiratory alkalosis | — |
| Renal | |
| Glomerular filtration rate | Increased (50%) |
| Renal plasma flow | Increased (50–75%) |
| Creatinine | Decreased |
| GI | |
| Gastric motility | Decreased |
| Alkaline phosphatase | Increased |
| Transaminases | Unchanged |
| LDH, amylase | Unchanged |
| Gallbladder contractility | Decreased |
| Biliary sludge/cholelithiasis | Increased |
| Endocrine | |
| Thyroid-binding globulin | Increased |
| $T_4$ | Increased |
| Total | Increased |
| Free | Unchanged |
| $T_3$ | Increased |
| TSH | Unchanged |
| Thyroid-releasing hormone | Unchanged |
| Prolactin | Increased |
| Cortisol | Increased |
| Aldosterone | Increased |

## SUGGESTED READING

Cunningham FB, Gant NF, Leveno KJ, et al., eds. *Williams obstetrics*, 21st ed. New York: McGraw-Hill, 2001.

**Prenatal Care**

*Guidelines for routine prenatal care*

## ROUTINE PRENATAL CARE
### Screening

Recommendations for routine screening are as follows:

### *Initial Prenatal Visit*

- Hgb and Hct
- Coomb's test
- Rh type
- Rubella titer
- VDRL or RPR (syphilis)
- HBsAg
- UA
- Gonorrhea and chlamydia
- Pap smear
- HIV
- Consider: Hgb electrophoresis, PPD, genetic counseling

### *16–18 Wks*

- Maternal serum screening (alpha-fetoprotein)
- U/S

### *26–28 Wks*

- 1-hr glucose challenge test
- Coombs' test
- Hgb and Hct

### *28 Wks*

- RhoGAM if Rh (–)

### *32–36 Wks*

- Hgb and Hct
- Gonorrhea and chlamydia
- VDRL or RPR
- Group B *Streptococcus* culture

### Prenatal Visit Intervals

- <28 wks: q4wks
- 28–36 wks: q2wks
- >36 wks: q1wk

### Maternal Weight Gain

- Underweight: 28–40 lbs
- Normal weight: 25–35 lbs
- Overweight: 15–25 lbs

### Folic Acid Supplementation

- General population: 0.4 mg/d
- Previous child with neural tube defect: 4.0 mg/d
- Trauma/maternal fetal hemorrhage
  - RhoGAM if Rh (–)
- Postpartum
  - RhoGAM: if mother Rh (–) and fetus Rh (+)
  - MMR vaccine: if mother rubella nonimmune

### IMMUNIZATIONS
See Table 3-1.

## TABLE 3-1.
## IMMUNIZATIONS DURING PREGNANCY

| Vaccine | Indications |
| --- | --- |
| **Live virus vaccines** | |
| MMR | Contraindicated |
| Varicella zoster | Contraindicated |
| Yellow fever | Contraindicated except if exposure to yellow fever virus possible |
| Poliomyelitis | No longer recommended even with risk of exposure |
| **Inactivated virus vaccines** | |
| Hepatitis A | Used extensively without adverse fetal effects |
| Hepatitis B | Not contraindicated |
| Influenza | Administer for those in second or third trimester during influenza season for patients with chronic conditions |
| Japanese encephalitis | Weigh risk of disease against possible vaccine benefits |
| Enhanced poliomyelitis | Risk of exposure |
| Rabies | Substantial risk of exposure |
| **Live bacterial vaccines** | |
| Typhoid (Ty21a) | Should reflect actual risk of disease and probable benefits of vaccine |
| **Inactivated bacterial vaccines** | |
| Cholera | Should reflect actual risk of disease and probable benefits of vaccine |
| Typhoid | Should reflect actual risk of disease and probable benefits of vaccine |
| Plague | Selective vaccination of exposed persons |
| Meningococcal | Only in unusual outbreaks |
| Pneumococcal | For women in all high-risk categories |
| *Haemophilus influenzae* (type B conjugate) | Only for high-risk women |
| Lyme | Safety has not been established |

(*continued*)

**TABLE 3-1.
(CONTINUED)**

| Vaccine | Indications |
| --- | --- |
| Toxoids | |
| Tetanus-diphtheria | Lack of primary series or no booster within past 10 yrs |
| Immune globulins | |
| Pooled or hyperim-mune | Exposure or anticipated unavoidable exposure to measles, hepatitis A, hepatitis B, rabies, or tetanus |

Reprinted from Gellin BG, Curlin GT, Rabinovich NR, et al. Adult immunization: principles and practice. *Adv Intern Med* 1999;44:327–352, with permission.

# Preterm Labor

*Preterm labor is a major cause of neonatal morbidity*

## DEFINITIONS

- Preterm labor (PTL): labor before 37 wks manifested by regular uterine contractions (q5–8mins) accompanied by cervical change [1].

- Cervical incompetence: cervical change in the absence of uterine activity.

## RISK FACTORS

See Table 4-1.

## HISTORY

- Contractions (duration, intensity)

- PTL risk factors

- Recent intercourse

- Sources of infection

- History of PROM

## PHYSICAL EXAM

- Vital signs (fever, tachycardia)

- Fundal tenderness, CVA tenderness

- Speculum exam (wet prep, rule out PROM) (see Chap. 5, Premature Rupture of Membranes)

- Cervical exam (dilation, effacement)

## DIAGNOSTIC EVALUATION

- Cervical length predicts risk of PTL

  - Cervical length <2.5 cm before 32 wks is associated with higher risk of preterm birth [2].

- Fetal fibronectin (fFN): glycoprotein involved in cell matrix adhesion

  - fFN obtained from cervical swab at time of speculum exam (before digital exam)

  - Negative fFN is strong predictor that preterm birth will not occur in next 2 wks

## TABLE 4-1.
## RISK FACTORS FOR PRETERM LABOR

Previous preterm delivery (17–37% recurrence)

Multiple gestations (10% of all preterm births)

Extremes of age (<18 or >40)

Infection (STDs, chorioamnionitis, systemic)

   Group B beta-hemolytic streptococcus

   *Neisseria gonorrhea*

   *Chlamydia trachomatis*

   *Trichomonas vaginalis*

   *Ureaplasma urealyticum*

   *Treponema pallidum*

   Bacterial vaginosis

Nonwhite race

Low socioeconomic status

Previous second trimester loss

Polyhydramnios

Uterine malformations

Substance abuse

   Drugs

   Tobacco

Preterm prolonged PROM

Cervical incompetence

---

- • Positive results of fFN are less useful [3]
- • Home uterine contraction monitoring: ineffective in preventing preterm birth
- • Lab: CBC, urine culture, urine drug screen, cervical swab for gonorrhea and chlamydia
- • Fetal assessment: nonstress test or biophysical profile, estimated fetal weight, amniotic fluid index

## MANAGEMENT
- • Treatment is aimed at delaying delivery until after 34 wks.
- • **IV fluid** hydration is the initial treatment.

- D5 half normal saline, 125 cc/hr
- Monitor fluids in patients receiving tocolytics (prevent pulmonary edema).
- **Tocolytics** are often used before 34 wks, although they have not been shown to improve neonatal survival or outcome (Table 4-2).
  - Contraindications for tocolysis: persistent fetal distress, chorioamnionitis, abruptio placentae, severe preeclampsia, documented fetal lung maturity, intrauterine fetal demise.
- **Corticosteroids** between 24 and 34 wks decrease neonatal mortality, respiratory distress syndrome, and intraventricular hemorrhage [4].
  - Betamethasone (Celestone), 12 mg IM × 2 (24 hrs apart)
  - Dexamethasone (Decadron), 6 mg IM × 4 (12 hrs apart)
  - Do not give multiple courses
- **Antibiotics:** not indicated unless PROM occurs with PTL.
  - If delivery appears imminent, prophylaxis against group B beta-hemolytic streptococcus warranted.
- **Unproven therapy**
  - Bed rest
  - Avoidance of intercourse
  - Prophylactic cerclage (only if history of cervical incompetence)
  - Treatment of bacterial vaginosis

**TABLE 4-2.**
**COMMONLY USED TOCOLYTICS**

| Drug | Dose | Side effects | Contraindications | Notes |
|------|------|--------------|-------------------|-------|
| $MgSO_4$ | 6 g IV load, then 2–3 g/hr | Flushing, headache, vision changes, nausea, lethargy, constipation, urinary retention, pulmonary edema, respiratory depression, cardiac arrest, tetany, hypotension | Hypocalcemia, myasthenia gravis, renal failure, heart block | Mg level: 7–10: loss of deep tendon reflexes; 10–12: respiratory depression; >12: cardiac arrest, hypotension, arrhythmias |
| Indomethacin | 50–100 mg PR, then 25 mg PO q6h × 48 hrs | Hepatitis, renal failure, GI bleeding, oligohydramnios, constriction of fetal ductus arteriosus, increased neonatal intraventricular hemorrhage, and necrotizing enterocolitis | Drug-induced asthma, CAD, GI bleed, oligohydramnios, renal failure, fetal cardiac/renal anomaly | Monitor amniotic fluid index<br>Used for brief periods (<48 hrs)<br>Avoid after 32 wks |
| Nifedipine | 10–20 mg PO q4–6h; can load 10 mg q20mins × 3 | Flushing, headache, nausea, hypotension, hepatotoxicity | Liver disease | — |
| Terbutaline | IV: 0.125 mg/hr, titrate to contractions q10–30mins (max, 0.25mg/hr)<br>0.25 mg IM/SQ q1–4h<br>2.5–7.5 mg PO q2–6h<br>Pump: 0.3–0.5 mg/hr with bolus of 0.25 mg prn | Palpitations, flushing, restlessness, hyperglycemia, hypokalemia, hypotension, pulmonary edema, arrhythmias, MI | Cardiac disease, arrhythmia, poorly controlled diabetes mellitus, HTN, thyrotoxicosis | Hold if maternal pulse >130 bpm or SBP <80–90 mm Hg |

## REFERENCES

1. American College of Obstetricians and Gynecologists. Assessment of risk factors for preterm birth. *ACOG Practice Bulletin 31.* Washington, DC: ACOG, 2001.

2. Iams JD, Goldenberg RL, Meis PJ, et al. National Institutes of Child Health and Human Development Maternal-Fetal Medicine Unit Network: The length of the cervix and risk of premature delivery. *N Engl J Med* 1996;334:567.

3. Lockwood CJ, Senyei AE, Dische MR. Fetal fibronectin in cervical and vaginal secretions as a predictor of preterm delivery. *N Engl J Med* 1991;325:669.

4. Collaborative Group on Antenatal Steroid Therapy. Effect of antenatal dexamethasone administration on the prevention of respiratory distress syndrome. *Am J Obstet Gynecol* 1981;141:276.

# 5 Premature Rupture of Membranes

*PROM often precedes preterm labor*

## INTRODUCTION

- **PROM:** membrane rupture before the onset of labor [1].

- **Preterm PROM:** membrane rupture before 37 wks' gestation.

- **Prolonged PROM:** rupture of membranes for >12 hrs (some references use 18 or 24 hrs).

- PROM at term is usually accompanied by labor within 24 hrs.

- Maternal complications include intraamniotic infection, preterm labor, cord prolapse, and abruptio placentae.

## RISK FACTORS

See Table 5-1.

## HISTORY

- Gush or leakage of fluid.

- "Bloody show" and contractions may be present.

## PHYSICAL EXAM

- Speculum exam: pH testing (alkaline), ferning, cervical cultures, wet prep

- Digital exam: contraindicated in PROM (increases risk of infection)

- Vaginal pool (obtain sample of amniotic fluid pool if present for fetal lung maturity)

## DIAGNOSTIC EVALUATION

- U/S for amniotic fluid index

- Dye test (PROM suspected but unconfirmed)

  - 1 mL of indigo carmine in 9 mL normal saline instilled by amniocentesis

  - Positive if blue dye seen on vaginal tampon (confirms PROM)

- Fetal evaluation: U/S for weight, presentation, placenta location

## TABLE 5-1.
## RISK FACTORS FOR PRETERM PREMATURE RUPTURE OF MEMBRANES

| | |
|---|---|
| Intrauterine infection | Preterm labor |
| Low socioeconomic status | Prior preterm delivery |
| STDs | Smoking |
| Cervical conization | Vaginal bleeding |
| Polyhydramnios | Cerclage |
| Multiple gestation | |

## MANAGEMENT

Patients with preterm PROM may be delivered or managed expectantly. Either strategy is acceptable for patients at 32–34 wks.

- **Delivery:**

  - Chorioamnionitis, nonreassuring fetal status, abruptio placentae, or confirmed fetal lung maturity should undergo induction of labor.

  - Patients at or beyond 34 wks are often delivered [2].

- **Expectant management:** bed rest and fetal monitoring

## TABLE 5-2.
## ANTIBIOTIC REGIMENS FOR PREMATURE RUPTURE OF MEMBRANES

**Regimen 1**

Ampicillin (Omnipen, Principen, Totacillin), 2 g IV q6h × 48 hrs

Erythromycin (E-Mycin, E.E.S., Ery-Tab, Eryc, EryPed, Ilosone), 250 mg IV q6h × 48 hrs, then

Amoxicillin (Amoxil, Biomox, Polymox, Trimox, Wymox), 500 mg PO tid × 5 d

Erythromycin (E-Mycin, E.E.S., Ery-Tab, Eryc, EryPed, Ilosone), 500 mg PO bid × 5 d

**Regimen 2**

Ampicillin/sulbactam (Unasyn), 1.5–3.0 mg IV q6h, then

Amoxicllin/clavulanate (Augmentin), 500–875 mg PO bid

- **Patients ≤32 wks' gestation**

  - Deliver if chorioamnionitis, placental abruption, or fetal distress occur.

  - Corticosteroids administered for PROM at 24–32 wks to decrease risk of respiratory distress syndrome.

  - Tocolytics may be given until corticosteroids administered.

  - Antibiotics prolong latency period and decrease risk of chorioamnionitis and neonatal sepsis (Table 5-2) [3].

## REFERENCES

1. American College of Obstetricians and Gynecologists. Premature rupture of membranes. *ACOG Practice Bulletin 1*. Washington, DC: ACOG, 1998.
2. Cox SM, Leveno KJ. Intentional delivery versus expectant management with preterm ruptured membranes at 30–34 weeks' gestation. *Obstet Gynecol* 1995;86:875–879.
3. Mercer BM, Miodovnik M, Thurnau GR, et al. Antibiotic therapy for reduction of infant morbidity after preterm premature rupture of the membranes: a randomized controlled trial. *JAMA* 1997;278:989–995.

# 6  Preeclampsia and Eclampsia

*Preeclampsia is a major cause of maternal morbidity*

## INTRODUCTION

- Hypertensive disorders complicate 6–8% of pregnancies.
- HTN is defined as a sustained SBP >140 mm Hg or a DBP >90 mm Hg [1, 2] (Table 6-1).

## EPIDEMIOLOGY

- Risk factors for preeclampsia: nulliparity, advanced age, black race, family history of preeclampsia, chronic HTN, chronic renal disease, DM, multiple gestations, and antiphospholipid antibody syndrome [3].

### Pathophysiology

- Etiology uncertain.
- Endothelial dysfunction and arterial vasospasm contribute to multi-system end-organ dysfunction (Table 6-2).

### History

- Neurologic symptoms (headache, scotomata, blurry vision, seizures)
- Edema
- Right upper quadrant pain (swelling of hepatic capsule)

### Physical Exam

- Vital signs (HTN)
- Edema
- Neurologic exam (hyperreflexia)
- Pulmonary exam (pulmonary edema)
- Cervical exam

### Diagnostic Evaluation

- CBC (hemoconcentration, thrombocytopenia)
- Uric acid, creatinine (elevated secondary to decreased GFR)

### TABLE 6-1.
### CLASSIFICATION OF HTN IN PREGNANCY

**Preeclampsia:** a pregnancy-specific syndrome observed after the 20th wk of pregnancy with SBP >140 mm Hg or DBP >90 mm Hg, accompanied by significant proteinuria (0.3 g in 24-hr specimen)

**Eclampsia:** preeclampsia accompanied by seizures that cannot be attributed to other causes

**Gestational HTN:** BP elevation detected after midpregnancy without proteinuria

**Chronic HTN:** HTN before the 20th wk of pregnancy or before pregnancy

**Hemolysis, elevated liver enzymes, and low platelet count (HELLP) syndrome:** subset of preeclampsia consisting of hemolysis, elevated liver enzymes, and low platelets

Adapted from the National Heart, Lung, and Blood Institute Report of the Working Group on Research on Hypertension in Pregnancy. *Am J Obstet Gynecol* 2000;183:S1–S22.

- Aminotransferases (elevated)

- 24-hr urine collection for protein and creatinine clearance

- Fetal assessment: nonstress test, estimated fetal weight, amniotic fluid index

### MANAGEMENT

- **Delivery is the only cure for preeclampsia.**

### TABLE 6-2.
### ORGAN SYSTEM EFFECTS OF PREECLAMPSIA

| System | Dysfunction |
| --- | --- |
| Cardiovascular | Increased cardiac output, systemic vasospasm |
| Hematologic | Hemoconcentration (intravascular volume contraction), thrombocytopenia (microangiopathic hemolysis) |
| Renal | Proteinuria, increased uric acid and creatinine (decreased GFR), extracellular volume expansion |
| Neurologic | Headaches, vision changes, hyperreflexia, seizures, blindness (occipital lobe edema) |
| Pulmonary | Pulmonary edema, ARDS |
| Hepatic | Elevated aminotransferases, subcapsular hematoma and hepatic rupture (periportal hemorrhage) |
| Fetal | Intrauterine growth rate, oligohydramnios (decreased uteroplacental perfusion) |

## Mild Preeclampsia

- Gestational age >37 wks: delivery.

- Gestational age <37 wks or patients with an unfavorable cervix may be temporized on bed rest.

- Worsening disease mandates delivery.

- $MgSO_4$ (as described under Magnesium) during labor [4].

- Monitor symptoms, urine protein, CBC, aminotransferases, and nonstress test.

## Severe Preeclampsia

- Gestational age >34 wks: delivery.

- Gestational age <34 wks: trial of observation and bed rest to temporize the disease and allow administration of corticosteroids.

- Worsening disease mandates delivery.

- Monitor urine output, pulmonary status, symptoms.

- Follow CBC, platelet count, urine protein, BP.

- Continuous fetal monitoring; follow fetal weight and amniotic fluid index.

- $MgSO_4$ as described under Magnesium.

## Eclampsia

- Maternal stabilization ($O_2$, IV access, protect airway).

- $MgSO_4$ as described under Magnesium.

- Valium, 10 mg IV, if further seizures while on $MgSO_4$.

- Continuous fetal monitoring.

- Delivery: may attempt vaginal delivery, but if fetal distress develops, c-section.

## HELLP Syndrome

- Delivery.

- $MgSO_4$ as described under Magnesium.

## Magnesium

- Administer $MgSO_4$ (4 g IV load, then 2 g/hr) to prevent seizures when delivery is indicated.

- $MgSO_4$ is superior to other anticonvulsants for seizure prophylaxis [5].

## Antihypertensives

- Administered if SBP is >160 mm Hg or DBP is >105 mm Hg.

- Hydralazine (Apresoline), 5–10 mg IV q20mins.

- Labetalol (Normodyne, Trandate), 20 mg IV followed by 40 mg in 10 mins, then 80 mg q10mins to a max of 220 mg.

- Sodium nitroprusside (Nipride), 0.25 µg/kg/min IV to a max of 5 mg/kg/min (requires central hemodynamic monitoring).

### Anesthesia

- Administer conduction anesthesia with care to prevent hypotension.

- Carefully monitor input and output.

### Prevention

- Aspirin (60–81 mg) may be of value in selected women at high risk for developing preeclampsia.

- Increased risk of abruptio placentae [6].

- Calcium (2 g/d) may reduce the risk of preeclampsia in selected populations.

- Vitamin E (400 IU) and ascorbic acid (1 g/d) have shown benefit in prophylaxis of preeclampsia in small trials.

### REFERENCES

1. National Heart, Lung, and Blood Institute Report of the Working Group on Research on Hypertension in Pregnancy. *Am J Obstet Gynecol* 2000;183:S1–S22.

2. American College of Obstetricians and Gynecologists. Diagnosis and management of preeclampsia and eclampsia. *ACOG Practice Bulletin 242*. Washington, DC: ACOG, 2002.

3. Sibai BM, Lindheimer M, Hauth J, et al. Risk factors for preeclampsia, abruptio placentae, and adverse neonatal outcomes among women with chronic hypertension. National Institute of Child Health and Human Development Network of Maternal-Fetal Medicine Units. *N Engl J Med* 1998;339:667–671.

4. The Magpie Trial Collaborative Group. Do women with preeclampsia, and their babies, benefit from magnesium sulphate? The Magpie Trial: a randomised placebo-controlled trial. *Lancet* 2002;359:1877–1890.

5. The Eclampsia Trial Collaborative Group. Which anticonvulsant for women with eclampsia? Evidence from the Collaborative Eclampsia Trial. *Lancet* 1995;345:1455–1463.

6. Sibai BM, Caritis SN, Thom E, et al. Prevention of preeclampsia with low-dose aspirin in healthy, nulliparous pregnant women. *N Engl J Med* 1993;329:1213–1218.

# 7

# Chronic Hypertension

*Careful blood pressure monitoring is mandatory throughout pregnancy*

## INTRODUCTION

- Chronic HTN: HTN preceding pregnancy or developing before 20 wks' gestation
- 5% of pregnancies
- Classification: severe if SBP >180 mm Hg or if DBP >110 mm Hg

## PATHOPHYSIOLOGY

- Fetal effects: intrauterine growth rate, prematurity, fetal distress, oligohydramnios, fetal demise
- Maternal effects: superimposed preeclampsia (50%), placental abruption, worsening HTN, CNS hemorrhage, cardiac decompensation, renal deterioration, increased rate of c-section

## PHYSICAL EXAM

- Vital signs (BP)
- Cervical exam
- Fundal height (monitor fetal growth)

## DIAGNOSTIC EVALUATION

- Search for end-organ damage
- Cardiac: ECG, echocardiography
- Renal: U/S, urine sediment, creatinine clearance, and total protein
- Visual: ophthalmologic exam
- Lab: BUN, creatinine, 24-hr urine for protein and creatinine clearance
- U/S at 18–20 wks and again at 28–32 wks to identify intrauterine growth rate
- Antenatal monitoring: nonstress tests (weekly or twice weekly beginning at 28–36 wks)

## MANAGEMENT

- Antihypertensive agents have been associated with decreased uteroplacental perfusion and low birth weight.

- Perform delivery at term unless other obstetric concerns arise.

### Mild Chronic Hypertension

- Antihypertensives not instituted.

- Consider dose reduction for patients already on medication.

### Severe Chronic Hypertension

- Begin antihypertensive medication.

- Goal is to reduce BP to the mild range.

- Antihypertensives

  - First-line agents

  - Methyldopa (Aldomet), 250 mg PO bid/tid (max, 3000 mg/d)

  - Labetalol (Normodyne, Trandate), 100 mg PO bid (max, 2400 mg/d)

  - Nifedipine (Procardia, Adalat), 10 mg PO tid (max, 120 mg/d)

- **ACE inhibitors are contraindicated.**

- Diuretics may be used but are second-line therapy.

## SUGGESTED READING

American College of Obstetricians and Gynecologists. Chronic hypertension in pregnancy. *ACOG Practice Bulletin 29*. Washington, DC: ACOG, 2001.

Sibai BM. Chronic hypertension in pregnancy. *Obstet Gynecol* 2002;100:369–377.

# 8

# Isoimmunization

*Type and screen all pregnant women*

## DEFINITION

- Isoimmunization: development of maternal antibodies to fetal antigens expressed on fetal RBCs in the maternal circulation [1].

## PATHOPHYSIOLOGY

- Maternal IgG antibodies cross the placenta, bind fetal RBCs, and cause hemolysis.

- Severe hemolysis results in fetal anemia with congestive heart failure, extramedullary hematopoiesis, hyperbilirubinemia, and kernicterus.

- Hydrops fetalis results when ascites, pleural effusions, pericardial effusions, and cerebral edema develop.

## IMMUNOLOGY

- Most common antigen: D (Rh) antigen.

- If mother D (−) and infant D (+), maternal antibodies may be produced, cross placenta, and interact with fetal RBCs.

- Magnitude of antibody response increases with each subsequent pregnancy.

- Other antigens that result in isoimmunization: Kell, E, c, C.

- Anti–Lewis IgM antibodies will not result in isoimmunization.

## HISTORY

Obstetric history (previous pregnancies with isoimmunization)

## DIAGNOSTIC EVALUATION

- See Table 8-1.

- **Rh typing** and antibody screen with indirect Coombs' test.

- **Paternal testing:** if the father is negative for the antigen, no further evaluation needed.

- **Antibody titers:** if >1:16, amniocentesis or cordocentesis.

- **Amniocentesis:** determine optical density (OD) at 450 nm (ΔOD 450) by spectrophotometry.

**TABLE 8-1.**
**DIAGNOSIS OF ISOIMMUNIZATION**

| | |
|---|---|
| **Antibody titer** | |
| <1:16 | Follow antibody titers |
| >1:16 | Amniocentesis or percutaneous umbilical blood sampling |
| **Amniocentesis (D ocular density 450)** | |
| Liley zone I | Repeat amniocentesis in 3–4 wks |
| Liley zone II | Repeat amniocentesis in 1–4 wks |
| | Follow D ocular density 450 trend in zone II |
| Liley zone III | Delivery or intrauterine transfusion |
| **Percutaneous umbilical sampling** | |
| Hct >25% | Monitor |
| Hct <25% | Intrauterine transfusion |

- $\Delta$OD 450 is an indirect assessment of amniotic fluid bilirubin.
- $\Delta$OD 450 value is plotted on the Liley graph (Fig. 8-1) to attempt to predict fetal outcome [2].

- **Percutaneous umbilical cord blood sampling**
  - Determine if fetus possesses the antigen to which the mother is producing antibodies.
  - Also used to measure fetal Hct.
- **U/S**
  - Hydropic fetuses display placental enlargement, ascites, pleural and pericardial effusions, polyhydramnios.
  - Serial U/S can be performed to evaluate worsening hydrops.
- **Middle cerebral artery velocity**
  - Measured by Doppler U/S.
  - Increased middle cerebral artery velocity correlated with moderate to severe fetal anemia [3].

## MANAGEMENT
- Serial amniocentesis, percutaneous umbilical blood sampling, and U/S detect evidence of worsening hydrops fetalis.

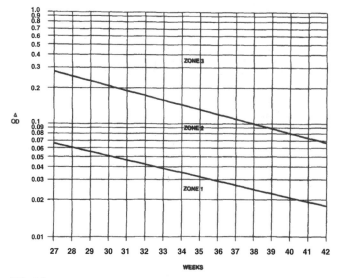

**FIG. 8-1.**
Liley graph. (Adapted from Liley AW. Liquor amnii analysis in the management of pregnancy complicated by rhesus sensitization. *Am J Obstet Gynecol* 1961;82:1359–1370.)

- Liley zone I or low zone II: delivery at term.
- Upper Liley zone II: delivery at 36–38 wks
- Liley zone III: transfusion or delivery

### Intrauterine Transfusion

- Performed if fetal Hct is <25% on percutaneous umbilical blood sampling or if the ΔOD 450 is in zone III and fetus is remote from delivery.
- Most commonly performed by percutaneous umbilical blood sampling.
- Transfused RBCs should be type O, Rh (–), CMV negative, washed, and birradiated.
- 30–100 mL blood may be transfused.
- Repeat transfusion may be required in 7–14 d.
- Mortality from intrauterine transfusion is 4–9%.
- Availability of neonatologists essential at time of delivery.

## REFERENCES

1. American College of Obstetricians and Gynecologists. Management of isoimmunization in pregnancy. *ACOG Educational Bulletin 227*. Washington, DC: ACOG, 1996.
2. Liley AW. Liquor amnii analysis in the management of pregnancy complicated by rhesus sensitization. *Am J Obstet Gynecol* 1961; 82:1359–1370.
3. Mari G, et al. Noninvasive diagnosis by Doppler ultrasonography of fetal anemia due to maternal red-cell alloimmunization. *N Engl J Med* 2000;342:9–14.

# 9 Nonimmune Hydrops Fetalis

*A variety of disorders can cause nonimmune hydrops fetalis*

## INTRODUCTION

- Hydrops fetalis: excessive accumulation of fluid in at least 2 fetal body cavities.
- Incidence: 1 in 1500–4000.
- Mortality: 50%.
- Nonimmune hydrops: result of any non–antibody-mediated process that leads to hydrops.
- Immune hydrops: hemolysis of fetal RBCs by maternal IgG antibodies to fetal antigens.

## DIAGNOSTIC EVALUATION
### U/S

- Ascites
- Pericardial and pleural effusions
- Placental enlargement
- Anatomic survey for anomalies
- Polyhydramnios
- Multiple gestation

### Lab Evaluation

- Hemoglobin electrophoresis
- Indirect Coombs' test
- TORCH (**to**xoplasmosis, **r**ubella, **C**MV, **h**erpes simplex)
- Syphilis (VDRL or RPR)
- Kleihauer-Betke

### Cordocentesis

Done for fetal karyotype, Hgb, Hbg electrophoresis, and IgM against possible infectious agents.

**TABLE 9-1.**
**DIFFERENTIAL DIAGNOSIS OF NONIMMUNE HYDROPS FETALIS**

Cardiovascular (20–45%)

    Tachyarrhythmia

    Structural defects

Chromosomal anomalies (35%)

    Trisomy 21

    Turner syndrome

    Other trisomies

    Triploidy

Hematologic disorders (10–27%)

    Thalassemia

Multiple gestation (10%)

    Twin-twin transfusion

    Respiratory disorders

    GI disorders

    Genitourinary disorders

    Placental anomalies

    Medications

Infectious diseases (10%)

    Toxoplasmosis

    CMV

    Syphilis

    Rubella

    Parvovirus

Idiopathic (22%)

### Amniocentesis

For karyotype, $\Delta$OD 450

### DIFFERENTIAL DIAGNOSIS

See Table 9-1.

### TREATMENT

- Depends on etiology.

- If fetus is viable, delivery is often indicated.

- If delivery not undertaken, antepartum monitoring should be instituted.

- Intrauterine transfusion may be performed for anemia.

- Termination may be offered early in gestation.

- Antepartum assessment of fetal well-being requires frequent monitoring.

- Complications: preeclampsia, preterm labor, postpartum hemorrhage.

- Fetal prognosis is guarded and newborn treatment best accomplished in a tertiary center.

## SUGGESTED READING

Forouzan I. Hydrops fetalis: recent advances. *Obstet Gynecol Surv* 1997;52(2):130–138.

# 10 Multiple Gestations

*Most complications of pregnancy are more common in multiple gestations*

## INTRODUCTION

- **Dizygotic twins:** 2 sperm and 2 eggs

  - Rate varies by age, race, and heredity and is increased by fertility drugs.

- **Monozygotic twins:** division of single sperm and ovum

  - Rate constant worldwide at 1 in 250 births

- The time of division determines the amnionicity and chorionicity of monozygotic twins (Table 10-1).

## PERINATAL COMPLICATIONS

- **Prematurity:** twin pregnancies average 36–37 wks, triplets 32–33 wks, quadruplets 31 wks

- **Birth weight:** lags behind singleton gestations after 32 wks

  - Monitor fetal growth using serial U/S

- **Twin-twin transfusion syndrome:** results from abnormal vascular communications in placenta

  - Incidence: 5–15% of monochorionic twins

  - One twin (donor twin) characterized by anemia, oligohydramnios, and intrauterine growth retardation

  - Second twin (recipient twin) marked by polycythemia, heart failure, nonimmune hydrops

  - Manifests at 20–30 wks and can be associated with preterm labor

  - Investigational therapies: therapeutic amniocentesis for polyhydramnios, laser coagulation of vessels

- **Monoamniotic twins**

  - 40% survival rate secondary to cord entanglement and fetal demise

  - Most problems that complicate singleton pregnancies occur with higher frequency in multiple gestations.

## TABLE 10-1.
## MONOZYGOTIC TWINS

| Day of division | Chorionicity | Amnionicity | Incidence |
| --- | --- | --- | --- |
| <3 days | Dichorionic | Diamnionic | 30% |
| 4–8 days | Monochorionic | Diamnionic | 68% |
| 8–14 days | Monochorionic | Monoamnionic | 2% |
| >14 days | Conjoined twins | Conjoined twins | Rare |

- Preterm labor, preeclampsia, gestational diabetes, intrauterine growth retardation, hyperemesis gravidarum, and postpartum hemorrhage are increased.

## ANTEPARTUM MANAGEMENT

- **U/S** for diagnosis

  - Sex, membrane thickness, and the "twin peaks" sign are indicators of zygosity.

  - Anomaly scan at 18–20 wks.

  - Serial sonography to monitor growth, fluid volume, and presentation.

  - Growth discordance of >20% mandates increased surveillance.

- **Genetics:** chromosome analysis is offered for women aged ≥31 yrs with twins and women ≥28 yrs with triplets.

- **Diet:** calorie intake is increased by 300 kcal/d.

  - Women should obtain 60 mg of elemental iron.

  - Monitor for signs of preterm labor and preeclampsia.

  - Consider antenatal surveillance with nonstress tests.

## INTRAPARTUM MANAGEMENT

- Multifetal gestations are delivered in the OR with a double setup in place.

- First twin nonvertex presentation: c-section.

- Vertex-vertex twins (40–45%): delivered vaginally.

- Vertex-nonvertex presentations (35–40%): may be delivered vaginally, the second twin delivered by external version, internal podalic version or breech extraction.

- The interval between delivery is not critical if fetal well-being is reassuring.

## SUGGESTED READING

American College of Obstetricians and Gynecologists. Special problems of multiple gestation. *ACOG Educational Bulletin 253*. Washington, DC: ACOG, 1998.

Chervenak FA, D'Alton ME. Multiple gestation. *Semin Perinatol* 1995;19:341–434.

# 11 Intrauterine Growth Retardation

*Intrauterine growth retardation (IUGR) requires careful evaluation and follow-up*

## DEFINITIONS

- **IUGR:** fetal weight is less than expected (usually less than the tenth percentile, often less than the third percentile).
- **Small for gestational age:** infant with a birth weight < tenth percentile; most are normal.

## PATHOPHYSIOLOGY

- Classification based on head-to-abdominal circumference ratio (HC/AC)
- **Symmetric IUGR:** HC/AC near 1; often occurs early in gestation
- **Asymmetric IUGR:** HC/AC >1; often develops late in gestation

## HISTORY

- Risk factors for IUGR
- Past medical history

## PHYSICAL EXAM

- Fundal height

## DIAGNOSTIC EVALUATION

- Based on differential diagnosis
- Serial U/S (fetal growth, amniotic fluid index, and umbilical artery velocimetry) at 2- to 4-wk intervals
- Serology for congenital infections
- Karyotype (aneuploidy)

## DIFFERENTIAL DIAGNOSIS

See Table 11-1.

## MANAGEMENT

- Antepartum monitoring
- Nonstress test or biophysical profile (weekly or biweekly)

**TABLE 11-1.**
**DIFFERENTIAL DIAGNOSIS OF INTRAUTERINE**
**GROWTH RETARDATION**

| Maternal causes | Fetal causes | Placental causes |
|---|---|---|
| Medical conditions | Viral infections | Chorioangioma |
| Cardiopulmonary diseases | CMV | Vascular insufficiency |
| HTN | Varicella | |
| DM | Toxoplasma | |
| Renal disease | Syphilis | |
| Anemia | Chromosomal anomalies | |
| Vascular disease | Congenital malformations | |
| Teratogens | | |
| Alcohol | | |
| Tobacco | | |
| Cocaine | | |
| Multiple gestations | | |
| Malnutrition | | |

- Initiate at 30–34 wks

- Delivery for nonreassuring fetal status, severe oligohydramnios, and absent fetal growth

- Must be individualized

## REFERENCES

1. American College of Obstetricians and Gynecologists. Intrauterine growth restriction. *ACOG Practice Bulletin 12*. Washington, DC: ACOG, 2000.
2. Resnik R. Intrauterine growth restriction. *Obstet Gynecol* 2002; 99:490–496.

# 12 Congenital Infections

*Common congenital infections*

## INTRODUCTION

Common congenital infections are described below. In general, the earlier in gestation that a fetus is exposed to an infectious agent, the more severe the consequences.

## TOXOPLASMOSIS

| | |
|---|---|
| Microbiology | Parasite: *Toxoplasma gondii* |
| Transmission | Cat feces, undercooked meat, infected soil, insect contamination of food |
| Maternal manifestations | Asymptomatic (most common) |
| | Symptomatic (10–20%): cervical adenopathy, fever, myalgias, hepatosplenomegaly |
| Maternal diagnosis | Serology (serial IgM and IgG specimens 3 wks apart) |
| Vertical transmission | Transmission rates: first trimester (10–15%), second (25%), third (60%) |
| | More severe with early transmission |
| Fetal diagnosis | U/S (cerebral calcifications, IUGR, ventriculomegaly, microcephaly, ascites, hepatosplenomegaly) |
| | Percutaneous umbilical blood sampling (serology) or PCR (amniocentesis) |
| Perinatal manifestations | Most asymptomatic at birth |
| | Late sequelae (55–85%): chorioretinitis, hearing loss, mental retardation, rash, fever, hepatosplenomegaly, periventricular calcifications, seizures |
| Treatment | Acute maternal infection: spiramycin |
| | Fetal infection: spiramycin, pyrimethamine, sulfonamides, and folinic acid |
| Screening | Preconception IgG, IgM, screening during pregnancy not recommended |

## VARICELLA ZOSTER

| | |
|---|---|
| Microbiology | DNA herpesvirus |
| | Incubation 10–20 d |
| | Infectivity 48 hrs before rash until all lesions crusted over |
| | Latent in sensory ganglia |
| Transmission | Respiratory |
| Maternal manifestations | Primary: chickenpox maculopapular, vesicular rash |
| | Chickenpox complications: pneumonia, encephalitis |
| | Secondary: zoster with vesicular rash in dermatomal pattern |
| Maternal diagnosis | Clinical exam |
| | Varicella antigen in lesions |
| Vertical transmission | Only in first 20 wks (1–2% transmission rate) |
| Fetal diagnosis | U/S (hydrops, limb deformities, IUGR, echogenic bowel, microcephaly) |
| | Serology (percutaneous umbilical blood sampling) |
| Perinatal manifestations | Congenital: limb hypoplasia, chorioretinitis, microcephaly |
| | Neonatal varicella: high mortality from maternal chickenpox 5 d before or 48 hrs after birth |
| Treatment | Acute maternal infection: acyclovir (within 24 hrs of developing rash) |
| | Maternal infection 5 d before or 48 hrs after delivery; neonatal varicella zoster immunoglobulin to prevent neonatal varicella |
| Prevention | No history of chickenpox-varicella vaccine (delay pregnancy until 1 mo after vaccine) |
| | Varicella exposure: test mother for VZV antibody; if negative, administer varicella zoster immunoglobulin within 72 hrs of exposure |
| | ✳ Varicella vaccine: contraindicated during pregnancy |

## CYTOMEGALOVIRUS

| | |
|---|---|
| Microbiology | DNA herpesvirus |
| | Viremia 2–3 wks after infection |
| | Latent in host |
| Transmission | Blood, urine, saliva, sexual contact |

| | |
|---|---|
| Maternal manifestations | Asymptomatic (most common) |
| | Symptomatic (primary): fever, malaise, lymphocytosis, elevated liver function tests |
| | Recurrent infections: usually asymptomatic |
| Maternal diagnosis | Serology (serial IgM and IgG specimens 3 wks apart) |
| | PCR of infected fluid |
| Vertical transmission | More severe effects with early transmission |
| | Transmission rates: primary infection (30–40%), recurrent infection (0.15–2%) |
| | 10% of infants develop sequelae after primary infection |
| Fetal diagnosis | U/S (hydrops, echogenic bowel, bowel calcifications, ventriculomegaly) |
| | Serology (percutaneous umbilical blood sampling) |
| | Culture or PCR (amniotic fluid) |
| Perinatal manifestations | Death, neurologic sequelae, hearing loss |
| Treatment | None |
| Screening | Preconception IgG, IgM in at-risk women. Screening during pregnancy not recommended. |

## PARVOVIRUS B19

| | |
|---|---|
| Microbiology | DNA virus |
| | Infectious 5–10 d after exposure; not infectious after rash develops |
| Transmission | Respiratory, hand-to-mouth contact |
| Maternal manifestations | Adults: rash and arthropathy or asymptomatic |
| | Aplastic crisis (patients with hemoglobinopathies) |
| | Children: erythema infectiosum (fifth disease) |
| Maternal diagnosis | Serology (IgM rise) |
| Vertical transmission | More severe affects with early transmission (<20 wks) |
| Fetal diagnosis | U/S (hydrops) |
| | PCR (placenta, amniocentesis) |
| Perinatal manifestations | Spontaneous abortion, hydrops (aplastic crisis, myocarditis), fetal death *in utero* |

| | |
|---|---|
| Treatment | Maternal IgG titers for 3–4 wks after exposure to detect seroconversion |
| | If no seroconversion fetus is not at risk |
| | If seroconversion monitor fetus by U/S for 10 wks (hydrops unlikely to develop after 10 wks) |
| | If hydrops develops PUBS for possible intrauterine transfusion |
| Screening | Not recommended |

## HERPES SIMPLEX

| | |
|---|---|
| Microbiology | DNA virus |
| | 2 serotypes: HSV 1 and HSV 2 |
| Transmission | Sexual and direct contact |
| Maternal manifestations | Primary infections: genital vesicles and ulcers often with systemic symptoms, including fever and myalgias |
| | Nonprimary first episode: genital vesicles and ulcers often without systemic symptoms |
| | Recurrent episode: recurrence of genital vesicles and ulcers |
| | Women average 2–4 recurrences during pregnancy |
| Maternal diagnosis | Cell culture |
| Vertical transmission | Most often from shedding from lower genital tract at delivery |
| | Rarely transplacental |
| | Risk of transmission: primary infection (50%), recurrent infection (4–5%) |
| Perinatal manifestations | Localized disease: skin, eye, mouth |
| | CNS disease |
| | Disseminated disease |
| Antepartum treatment | Primary episode: antiviral therapy |
| | Recurrent episode: consider antiviral therapy after 36 wks |
| | See Chap. 53, Vulvovaginitis for antiviral regimens |
| Intrapartum treatment | Active lesions: c-section |
| | No active lesions: careful pelvic exam and vaginal delivery |
| Screening | Not recommended |

## RUBELLA

| | |
|---|---|
| Microbiology | Virus |
| Transmission | Respiratory |
| Maternal manifestations | Asymptomatic (25%) |
| | Rash |
| Maternal diagnosis | Serology (IgM or rise in IgG in acute and convalescent sera) |
| Vertical transmission | Risk of defects: 11–12 wks (33%), 13–14 wks (11%), 15–16 wks (24%), >16 wks (0%) |
| Fetal diagnosis | U/S |
| Perinatal manifestations | Congenital rubella syndrome: sensorineural deafness, cataracts, heart defects (patent ductus arteriosus, septal defects), meningoencephalitis, IUGR, thrombocytopenia, hepatitis, pneumonitis |
| Treatment | None |
| Prevention | Vaccinate all children 12–15 mos of age |
| | Vaccinate all rubella nonimmune women (except during pregnancy) |
| | If pregnant patient is rubella nonimmune, administer MMR postpartum |
| Screening | Antibody titer preconception or at first prenatal visit |

## SYPHILIS

| | |
|---|---|
| Microbiology | Spirochete: *Treponema pallidum* |
| | Incubation 10–90 d |
| Transmission | Sexual contact |
| Maternal manifestations | Primary syphilis: painless ulcer (chancre) persists for 2–6 wks |
| | Secondary syphilis (6–8 wks after chancre): condyloma lata (genital ulcerations), rash, adenopathy |
| | Tertiary syphilis: cardiovascular, neurologic, and gummatous disease |
| | Latent syphilis: serology positive in absence of clinical disease |
| | Early latent syphilis (<1 yr), late latent syphilis (>1 yr) |
| Maternal diagnosis | Screening: nontreponemal serology (VDRL or RPR) |
| | Confirmation: treponemal serology (MHA-TP, FTA-ABS) |

| | |
|---|---|
| | Lumbar puncture if neurologic signs |
| Vertical transmission | Only develops after 18 wks' gestation |
| Fetal diagnosis | U/S |
| | PCR (amniotic fluid) |
| Perinatal manifestations | Preterm labor, spontaneous abortion, placentomegaly |
| | Congenital syphilis |
| | Early manifestations (first 2 yrs): rhinitis (snuffles), mucocutaneous lesions, osteochondritis, hepatosplenomegaly, adenopathy, jaundice |
| | Late manifestations (after 2 yrs): interstitial keratitis, Clutton's joints (knee effusions), neurosyphilis |
| | Residual stigmata: Hutchinson's teeth, mulberry molars, frontal bossing, saddle nose, rhagades |
| Treatment | Primary/secondary/early latent: benzathine penicillin G, 2.4 million U IM × 1 |
| | Late latent/tertiary: benzathine penicillin G, 2.4 million U IM q wk × 3 |
| | If penicillin allergy: desensitization |
| Screening | VDRL or RPR preconception or at first prenatal visit |

## SUGGESTED READING

American College of Obstetricians and Gynecologists. Management of herpes in pregnancy. *ACOG Practice Bulletin 8.* Washington, DC: ACOG, 1999.

American College of Obstetricians and Gynecologists. Perinatal viral and parasitic infections. *ACOG Practice Bulletin 20.* Washington, DC: ACOG, 2000.

# 13 Third-Trimester Bleeding

*Bleeding during pregnancy requires immediate evaluation*

## HISTORY

- Bleeding (amount, duration): attempt to quantify amount of clots, pads soaked
- Contractions
- Abdominal pain
- History of bleeding disorder

## PHYSICAL EXAM

- Vital signs (hypotension, tachycardia, orthostatics)
- Gentle sterile speculum exam (quantify bleeding, rule out PROM, genital pathology)
- Digital exam (rule out PROM, vasa previa, and placenta previa before exam)

## DIFFERENTIAL DIAGNOSIS

- Placental abruption.
- Vasa previa.
- Genital tract laceration.
- Marginal sinus.
- Placenta previa.
- Labor with cervical change.
- See Table 13-1.

## DIAGNOSTIC EVALUATION

- U/S (rule out placenta previa, confirm viable intrauterine pressure, assess amniotic fluid index)
- Lab: CBC, PTT, PT, fibrinogen
- Kleihauer-Betke
- Type and cross
- *Gonorrhea* and *Chlamydia* cultures (cervicitis)

**TABLE 13-1.**
**DIFFERENTIAL DIAGNOSIS OF PLACENTAL ABRUPTION AND PLACENTA PREVIA**

| Characteristic | Placental abruption | Placenta previa |
| --- | --- | --- |
| Contractions | Present | Absent |
| Abdominal pain | Present | Absent |
| Fetal heart rate | Nonreassuring (decelerations and tachycardia) | Reassuring |
| Bleeding | Continuous | Usually resolves |
| Coagulopathy | Common | Infrequent |

- Fetal assessment: nonstress test, biophysical profile, estimated fetal weight, amniotic fluid index

## PLACENTAL ABRUPTION

- Separation of the placenta from the site of implantation before delivery
- 1 in 75–200 pregnancies

### Pathology

- Blood may escape through the cervix, remain concealed behind placenta, or drain into amniotic cavity.
- Complete (entire placenta separates) or partial (only part of the placenta separates).
- Risk factors: trauma, drugs (cocaine, tobacco), PROM, HTN, leiomyomas.

### Management

- Hemodynamics: correct hypovolemia with crystalloid, packed RBCs
- Fresh frozen plasma and platelets if coagulopathy
- Delivery: patients at term, with heavy bleeding, fetal distress, or hemodynamic instability
  - Emergent c-section
- Surveillance: preterm with small abruption and mild bleeding
- Complications: dessiminated intravascular coagulation, acute renal failure, and Couvelaire's uterus (blood in the uterine musculature)

## PLACENTA PREVIA

- Placenta near or overlying the internal os
- 1 in 200–250 pregnancies
- Increased risk for placenta accreta

### Pathology

- Total (complete) previa: placenta covers entire cervical os
- Partial previa: placenta partially covers cervical os
- Marginal previa: placental edge is within 2 cm of internal os
- Low-lying placenta: placenta in lower uterine segment but >2 cm from cervical os
- Most low-lying placentas detected on U/S resolve

### Risk Factors

- Advanced age, previous c-section, multiparity, previous placenta previa, prior induced abortion

### Diagnosis

- Painless vaginal bleeding
- First bleeding usually occurs in the second or third trimester and resolves

## MANAGEMENT

- Delivery: full term, unremitting bleeding
  - Usually c-section
- Bed rest and close observation: if bleeding subsides
  - Administer corticosteroids if premature (<32–34 wks)
  - Tocolysis with $MgSO_4$ considered
  - Delivery by c-section after fetal lung maturity documented
  - Outpatient bed rest considered in stable, compliant patients

## SUGGESTED READING

Cunningham FG, Gant NF, Leveno KJ, et al., eds. *Williams obstetrics,* 21st ed. New York: McGraw-Hill, 2001.

# 14 Abortion

*Spontaneous and elective abortion*

## SPONTANEOUS ABORTION

### Threatened Abortion

- Vaginal bleeding before 20 wks' gestation
- 50% will abort
- Evaluation
  - Rule out other causes of bleeding
  - U/S to confirm an intrauterine pregnancy and rule out ectopic pregnancy
- Management: RhoGAM if Rh (–), bed rest

### Incomplete Abortion

- Retained placenta after fetal expulsion
- Management: suction curettage if heavy bleeding, or may pass tissue spontaneously

### Complete Abortion

- All products of conception are spontaneously expelled

### Inevitable Abortion

- Cervical dilation with membrane rupture
- Management: expectant management or therapeutic abortion

### Missed Abortion

- Products of conception are not expelled after fetal death
- Management: expectant management or therapeutic abortion

## ELECTIVE ABORTION

- 1,360,000 therapeutic abortions performed in U.S. in 1996

### Suction Curettage

- Perform before 14 wks

- Most common procedure for first-trimester abortion
- Cervical dilation required
- Complications: uterine perforation, lacerations, incomplete fetal evacuation

### Dilation and Evacuation (D & E)

- Abortions after 13–16 wks
- Mechanical dilation of cervix followed by evacuation of fetal tissue
- Laminaria or synthetic osmotic dilators aid dilation
- Complications: uterine perforation, lacerations, incomplete fetal evacuation
- Uterotonics for uterine atony

### Mifepristone (RU-486)

- Progesterone antagonist [1]
- First-trimester abortions
- Administration described in Table 14-1
- Misoprostol also given to aid expulsion of the products of conception

### Misoprostol

- Prostaglandin $E_1$ analogue [2]
- Used alone or with mifepristone for first-trimester abortion
- Elective second-trimester terminations or induction of labor after fetal death *in utero* in second or third trimester

### TABLE 14-1.
### MIFEPRISTONE

| | |
|---|---|
| Administration | Mifepristone, 200 mg PO (day 1) |
| | Misoprostol, 200 μg PO × 2 tabs or 800 μg intravaginal (day 3) |
| | Confirm complete abortion (day 14) |
| Contraindications | Ectopic pregnancy, IUD, adrenal insufficiency, hemorrhagic disorder, coagulopathy, porphyria |
| Side effects | Vaginal bleeding, abdominal pain, nausea and vomiting, diarrhea |
| Success (complete expulsion) | <49 d: 92%; 50–56 d: 83%; 57–63 d: 77% |

- Side effects: vomiting, diarrhea
- Regimens:
  - 200–600 µg vaginally q12h (second-trimester abortion)
  - 400 µg vaginally q4h (second-trimester abortion)
  - 100 µg vaginally q12h (third-trimester induction)

## Other Techniques

- Intraamniotic infusion of saline or urea: used infrequently
- Hysterotomy: higher rate of complications; not used routinely

## REFERENCES

1. Grimes DA, Chaney EJ, Connell EB, et al. FDA approval of mifepristone: an overview. *Contraception Rep* 2000;11:4–12.
2. Goldberg AB, Greenberg MB, Darney PD. Misoprostol and pregnancy. *N Engl J Med* 2000;344:38–47.

# 15 Fetal Demise

*A thorough evaluation should be performed for fetal demise* in utero

## INTRODUCTION

- Fetal death rate 7.5/1000 in United States
- Fetal death *in utero* mandates thorough evaluation

## DIFFERENTIAL DIAGNOSIS

- Maternal diseases: poorly controlled diabetes, HTN, collagen vascular diseases, SLE with antiphospholipid antibodies, hemoglobinopathies
- Bacterial and viral infections: listeria monocytogenes, syphilis, CMV, rubella, toxoplasmosis, parvovirus B19
- Placental abruption
- Umbilical cord accident
- Fetomaternal hemorrhage
- Congenital anomalies and chromosomal abnormalities
- Drugs

## DIAGNOSTIC EVALUATION

- See Table 15-1.
- Chromosomal analysis: specimens of fetal skin, fascia lata, patellar tendon, or blood placed in genetic media, **not** formalin
- Pathology: placenta, infant inspected for abnormalities, and fetal autopsy

## MANAGEMENT

- Delivery: induction of labor with prostaglandins
- Grief: provide psychological counseling; allow parents opportunity to hold fetus
- Complications: disseminated intravascular coagulation if prolonged retained fetus
- Follow up: in 4–8 wks to review lab and pathology data

**TABLE 15-1.**
**DIAGNOSTIC EVALUATION OF FETAL DEMISE**

Lab

    VDRL

    Hbg A1C

    PT, PTT

    ANA

    CBC

    Anticardiolipin antibody

    Lupus anticoagulant

    Kleihauer-Betke

    Toxicology screen

    Hgb electrophoresis

Pathology

    Fetal autopsy

    Placenta

Karyotype

Serology

    CMV

    Toxoplasmosis

    Rubella

    Parvovirus B19

    Herpes simplex

## REFERENCE

1. Cunningham FB, Gant NF, Leveno KJ, et al., eds. *Williams obstetrics*, 21st ed. New York: McGraw-Hill, 2001.

# 16 Teratology

*Common teratogens*

## DRUGS
See Tables 16-1 and 16-2.

## RADIATION

- High dose (>25 rads): microcephaly, mental retardation, IUGR
- Greatest risk: between wks 8 and 15
- Larger doses teratogenic between wks 16 and 25
- No proved risk for fetuses <8 wks or >25 wks
- Doses of <5 rads produce no fetal abnormalities
- Fetal risk minimized by abdominal shielding
- Counseling: reassure mothers exposed to radiation that risk of fetal effects is small, especially at low doses and after 25 wks (Table 16-3)
- MRI and U/S: safe
- V/Q scans: minimal (50 mrad) fetal exposure
- Radioactive iodine: taken up by the fetal thyroid gland after 10–12 wks; absolutely contraindicated

## SUBSTANCES OF ABUSE

- Alcohol: fetal alcohol syndrome causing IUGR, postnatal growth deficiencies, mental retardation, behavioral disturbances, abnormal facies, heart and brain abnormalities
- Cocaine: maternal medical complications (MI, bowel infarction, HTN, and preeclampsia), placental abruption, and congenital anomalies
- Tobacco: low-birth-weight infants, placental abruption, and spontaneous abortions
- Marijuana: not associated with fetal anomalies
- Social work consultation should be obtained for referral for drug rehabilitation

## TABLE 16-1.
## FDA CLASSIFICATION OF MEDICATIONS

Category A: No fetal risks in human studies

Category B: No fetal risks in animal studies

Category C: Adverse effects in animal studies but no human data

Category D: Fetal risks but benefits of medication may outweigh risk

Category X: Fetal risks outweigh benefits

## TABLE 16-2.
## COMMON TERATOGENS

Antimicrobials

| | |
|---|---|
| Tetracycline/doxycycline | Yellow/brown tooth discoloration |
| Chloramphenicol | Gray baby syndrome: neonatal cyanosis, vascular collapse |
| Sulfonamides | Hyperbilirubinemia |
| Fluoroquinolones | Arthropathy (dog studies) |
| Ribavirin | Hydrocephalus, limb abnormalities |

**Generally considered safe:** penicillin, cephalosporins, aminoglycosides, clindamycin (Cleocin Oral, Cleocin T), nitrofurantoin (Furadantin, Macrobid, Macrodantin), and acyclovir (Zovirax)

Cardiovascular agents

| | |
|---|---|
| Beta blockers | IUGR (most commonly, atenolol) |
| ACE inhibitors | Renal anomalies, nephrotoxicity, oligohydramnios, pulmonary hypoplasia, IUGR |
| Thiazide diuretics | Neonatal thrombocytopenia |
| Anticoagulants: coumadin | Fetal warfarin syndrome (15–25% of those exposed): nasal hypoplasia, microcephaly, stippled vertebral and femoral epiphyses, spontaneous abortion, neonatal deaths |
| | Switch patients to heparin or LMWH before and during pregnancy (heparin and LMWH do not cross the placenta and are the anticoagulants of choice during pregnancy) |

*(continued)*

## TABLE 16-2.
## (CONTINUED)

Antiepileptics

| | |
|---|---|
| Phenytoin (Dilantin, Dilantin-125, Dilantin Infatabs, Dilantin Kapseals, Phenytek) | Fetal hydantoin syndrome: limb abnormalities, craniofacial defects, IUGR, mental retardation |
| Valproate (Depacon) | Craniofacial defects |
| Carbamazepine (Atretol, Depitol, Epitol, Tegretol) | Similar to phenytoin |
| | Patients already on antiepileptics are generally continued on their pregestational medications during pregnancy. Patients who have been free of seizures for several years may be given a trial of discontinuing their antiepileptics under the guidance of a neurologist before pregnancy. |

Analgesics

| | |
|---|---|
| Narcotics | Neonatal depression (administration near delivery) |
| NSAIDs | Premature closure of fetal ductus arteriosus after 34 wks |

Miscellaneous

| | |
|---|---|
| Vitamin A isomers (Accutane) | Craniofacial defects, heart defects, brain anomalies |
| Thalidomide | Exposure 27–30 d: upper extremity phocomelia; exposure 30–33 d: lower extremity phocomelia |
| Oral contraceptive pills | Not associated with fetal malformations |

.E 16-3
## ESTIMATED FETAL EXPOSURE FROM COMMON RADIOLOGIC STUDIES

| Procedure | Fetal exposure |
| --- | --- |
| Chest x-ray (2 view) | 0.02–0.07 mrad |
| Abdominal film (1 view) | 100 mrad |
| IV pyelogram | >1 rad |
| Hip film (1 view) | 200 mrad |
| Mammogram | 7–20 mrad |
| Barium enema/small bowel series | 2–4 rad |
| CT (head or chest) | <1 rad |
| CT (abdomen or lumbar spine) | 3.5 rad |
| CT pelvimetry | 250 mrad |

Reprinted from American College of Obstetricians and Gynecologists. *Guidelines for diagnostic imaging during pregnancy (Committee Opinion No. 158)*. Washington, DC:ACOG, 1995, with permission.

## SUGGESTED READING

American College of Obstetricians and Gynecologists. Guidelines for diagnostic imaging during pregnancy. *ACOG Committee Opinion 158*. Washington, DC: ACOG, 1995.

# 17

# Nausea and Vomiting in Pregnancy

*Nausea and vomiting (N/V) accompany most pregnancies*

## INTRODUCTION

- Affects 70–85% of gravid females.

- **Hyperemesis gravidarum:** severe form of N/V associated with inability to tolerate oral intake; >5% weight loss, ketonuria.

- **Pytalism:** increased salivation that contributes to dehydration.

## PATHOPHYSIOLOGY

- Etiology: uncertain.

- Elevated hCG may stimulate vomiting center in medulla oblongata.

- Onset: 5–6 wks with peak at 9 wks.

- Most symptoms resolve by 16 wks (rarely persists >20 wks).

- Usually worse in the morning but occurs all day.

- Odors may be triggers.

## HISTORY

- Abdominal pain, fever, and headache suggest an organic etiology.

## DIAGNOSTIC EVALUATION

- CBC, electrolytes

- UA (examine for ketonuria)

- Liver function tests (AST and ALT may be elevated, rarely >300 U/L)

- Bilirubin (usually <4 mg/dL)

- Amylase (may be up to 5 times normal)

- TSH (often decreased)

- U/S (evaluate gestational age; rule out molar gestation)

## DIFFERENTIAL DIAGNOSIS

See Table 17-1.

**TABLE 17-1.**
**DIFFERENTIAL DIAGNOSIS OF NAUSEA AND VOMITING**

| GI | Metabolic |
|---|---|
| Gastroparesis | Diabetic ketoacidosis |
| Gastroenteritis | Addison's disease |
| Achalasia | Hyperthyroidism |
| Cholelithiasis | Neurologic |
| Ileus | Pseudotumor cerebri |
| Intestinal obstruction | Vestibular lesions |
| Peptic ulcer disease | Migraine headaches |
| Pancreatitis | CNS neoplasm |
| Appendicitis | Miscellaneous |
| Hepatitis | Drug toxicity |
| Genitourinary | Preeclampsia |
| Pyelonephritis | Psychologic |
| Uremia | Trophoblastic disease |
| Ovarian torsion | Acute fatty liver of pregnancy |
| Nephrolithiasis | |
| Degenerating leiomyoma | |

Adapted from Herbert WN, et al. *Nausea and vomiting of pregnancy.*
Washington, DC: APGO, 2001.

## MANAGEMENT

- Hospitalization if electrolyte abnormalities or severe vomiting refractory to outpatient management.
- IV fluid hydration (initially normal saline boluses then D5 1/2 normal saline 125–150 cc/hr).
- Electrolyte replacement with IV potassium (40 mEq IV over 4 hrs) and magnesium ($MgSO_4$; 2 g IV).
- Dietary modification: frequent small meals, high carbohydrate/low-fat diets, protein-dominant diets, bland foods, small amounts of carbonated fluids.
- Avoid offensive odors.
- Antiemetics: vitamin $B_6$ or doxylamine (Unisom Nighttime Sleep-Aid) are first-line therapy (Table 17-2).

**TABLE 17-2.**
**ANTIEMETICS**

Vitamin $B_6$, 10–25 mg tid or qid PO

Doxylamine (Unisom), 12.5 mg tid or qid PO

Promethazine (Phenergan), 12.5–25 mg q4–6 PO/IM/PR

Meclizine (Antivert), 25–100 mg qd PO

Diphenhydramine (Dramamine), 50–75 mg q4–6h PO

Metoclopramide (Reglan), 5–10 mg q8h PO/IM/IV

Prochlorperazine (Compazine), 2.5–10 mg q3–4h PO/IM or 25 mg bid PR

Ondansetron (Zofran), 8 mg q12h PO/IM/IV

Methylprednisolone (Solu-Medrol), 16 mg q8h IV/PO × 3 d (taper over 2 wks)

- Alternative therapies: ginger, mint, orange (unproved), acupressure, psychotherapy.
- Enteral supplements or TPN if refractory.

**REFERENCE**

1. Herbert WN, Goodwin TM, Koren G, et al. Association of professors of gynecology and obstetrics educational series. *Nausea and vomiting of pregnancy.* Washington, DC: APGO, 2001.

# 18 Trauma in Pregnancy

*Maternal stabilization is the first priority*

## INTRODUCTION

- Trauma results in 1300–3900 fetal losses/yr.
- Major traumas: 40–50% fetal loss rate.
- Minor trauma: 1–5% incidence of fetal loss.

## MAJOR TRAUMA
### Blunt Abdominal Trauma

- Usually motor vehicle accident.
- Fetal loss often secondary to traumatic placental abruption.
- Direct fetal injury and uterine rupture less common.

### Pelvic Fractures

- Associated with large-volume retroperitoneal hemorrhage.

### Penetrating Trauma

- Gunshot or stab wound.
- Fetal demise from direct fetal or placental injury.

### Management

- Maternal stabilization is first priority.
- Fetal assessment after mother stabilized.
- Evaluation in Table 18-1.
- Give RhoGAM if mother is Rh (–).

## MINOR TRAUMA

- Falls and minor motor vehicle accidents.
- Maternal stabilization and fetal assessment as above.
- Traumatic placental abruption may still occur.
- Fetal heart rate and uterine contraction monitoring for 2–6 hrs.
- Contractions or fetal decelerations worrisome for placental abruption.

## TABLE 18-1.
## MANAGEMENT OF TRAUMA IN PREGNANCY

Maternal stabilization

    Primary survey (airway/breathing/circulation)

    Place two large-bore IV lines

    Lateral decubitus position (if no spinal injury/CPR)

    $O_2$ (nasal cannula or face mask)

    IV hydration (normal saline or lactated Ringer's)

    Vasopressors (if refractory hypotension)

    Secondary survey

    Imaging (CT/x-ray prn)

    Lab (CBC, PT, PTT, electrolytes)

Fetal assessment

    Electronic fetal monitoring/tocodynameter

    U/S (gestational age, viability)

    Cervical exam

    Speculum exam (premature rupture of membranes)

    Lab (Kleihauer-Betke)

- Give RhoGAM if mother Rh (–).

- Counseling: reassure mother that further complications are rare if no evidence of abruption or preterm labor in 4–6 hrs.

### PERIMORTEM CESAREAN SECTION

- Performed if cardiopulmonary arrest in the third trimester after 4–5 mins of resuscitative efforts.

- Improves maternal blood return and aids resuscitative efforts.

### SUGGESTED READING

American College of Obstetricians and Gynecologists. Obstetric aspects of trauma management. *ACOG Educational Bulletin 251.* Washington, DC: ACOG, 1998.

Katz VL, Dotter DJ, Droegemueller W. Perimortem cesarean delivery. *Obstet Gynecol* 1986;68:571–576.

# Medical Complications of Pregnancy

# 19          Asthma

*Asthma should be treated aggressively during pregnancy*

## INTRODUCTION

- Asthma in pregnancy associated with preterm birth, low-birth-weight infants, perinatal mortality, preeclampsia.

## PATHOPHYSIOLOGY

- Reversible airway obstruction secondary to airway hypersensitivity.

- Air trapping from bronchial wall edema, secretions, and mucus plugging.

- Triggers: infections, cold weather, allergens, dust or pollution, NSAIDs.

- In pregnancy, one-third of asthma patients improve, one-third worsen, and one-third stabilize.

## CLASSIFICATION

NIH classification of asthma and indications for pharmacotherapy (Table 19-1) [1].

## ANTEPARTUM MANAGEMENT

- See Table 19-2.

- Patient education, hydration, avoidance of triggers.

- Peak expiratory flow: does not change during pregnancy.

  - Measure at each visit.

- Immunizations: influenza vaccine after first trimester.

- Pharmacotherapy: see Tables 19-1 and 19-2.

- Continue medications during labor.

- Stress-dose steroids (hydrocortisone, 100 mg IV q8h) in labor and for 24 hrs postpartum if IV or PO steroids used peripartum.

- Antepartum monitoring: fetal activity assessment daily after 28 wks, weekly or biweekly nonstress tests beginning at 32–34 wks.

- Patients with severe persistent asthma are managed in conjunction with an asthma specialist.

## TABLE 19-1.
## NIH CLASSIFICATION OF ASTHMA

| Category | Symptoms | Lung function | Medications |
|---|---|---|---|
| Mild inter-mittent | <2/wk; brief exacerbations | $FEV_1$/ PEF >80% predicted; PEF variability <20% | prn beta$_2$-agonist |
| Mild persistent | >2/wk; <1 daily; exacerbations affect activity | $FEV_1$/PEF >80% predicted; PEF variability 20–30% | prn beta$_2$-agonist; single antiinflammatory agent (low-dose inhaled steroid, cromolyn, or nedocromil) |
| Moderate persistent | Daily symptoms; exacerbations >2/wk that affect activity | $FEV_1$/PEF 60–80% predicted; PEF variability >30% | Inhaled corticosteroid (medium dose) or long-acting beta$_2$-agonist |
| Severe persistent | Continued symptoms; limits activity; frequent exacerbations | $FEV_1$/PEF < 60% predicted; PEF variability >30% | Inhaled corticosteroid (high dose) and long-acting beta$_2$-agonist |

PEF, peak expiratory flow.
Adapted from National Asthma Education and Prevention Program. *Guidelines for the diagnosis and management of asthma.* Bethesda: National Institutes of Health, 1997.

## ACUTE EXACERBATIONS
### History

- Shortness of breath
- Chest tightness
- Wheezing
- Fever
- Cough

### Physical Exam

- General appearance, use of accessory muscles
- Vital signs: tachycardia, tachypnea, pulsus paradoxus
- Pulse oximetry: hypoxia
- Pulmonary auscultation: wheezes, prolonged expiratory phase

**TABLE 19-2.**
**ASTHMA MEDICATIONS**

| Medication | Dosage |
| --- | --- |
| Short-acting beta$_2$-agonists | |
|    Albuterol (Ventolin) | Nebulized 2.5 mg (0.5-mL solution with 2–3 mL NS) prn |
| | MDI 2 puffs q 4 prn |
| Long-acting beta$_2$-agonists | |
|    Salmeterol (Serevent) | MDI 2 puffs bid |
|    Albuterol (sustained release) | 4 mg tablet q12h |
| Anticholinergics | |
|    Ipratropium (Atrovent) | MDI 2–3 puffs qid (nebulized tid/qid) |
|    Cromolyn (Intal) | MDI 2–4 puffs tid/qid |
|    Nedocromil (Tilade) | 2 puffs qid |
| Methylxanthines | |
|    Theophylline | 10 mg/kg/d PO (300 max initial dose) |
| Leukotriene mediators | |
|    Zafirlukast (Accolate) | 40 mg qd PO |
|    Montelukast (Singulair) | 10 mg qpm PO |
| Inhaled corticosteroids | |
|    Beclomethasone (Vanceril) | 2 puffs tid |
|    Flunisolide (AeroBid) | 2–4 puffs bid |
|    Fluticasone (Flovent) | 2–4 puffs bid |
|    Triamcinolone (Azmacort) | 2 puffs tid–qid |
| Systemic corticosteroids | |
|    Methylprednisolone | 60–80 mg IV q6–8h |
|    Prednisone | 60–120 mg/d divided doses, tapered |

## Diagnostic Evaluation

- ABG (hypoxia)
- Chest x-ray (rule out pneumonia)
- Nonstress test or biophysical profile

- U/S: fetal growth
- Differential diagnosis
- Pneumonia
- Bronchitis
- Pulmonary embolism
- Pulmonary edema
- Peripartum cardiomyopathy
- Management
- $O_2$: nasal canula or face mask titrate saturation >95%
- Beta$_2$-agonists: nebulized treatment, then MDI, repeat q20–30mins prn
- Hospitalization: if symptoms do not improve after beta-agonist treatment
- Corticosteroids: for patients who require hospitalization

## REFERENCE

1. National Asthma Education and Prevention Program. *Guidelines for the diagnosis and management of asthma.* Bethesda: National Institutes of Health, 1997.

# 20 Diabetes Mellitus

*Diabetes causes serious neonatal morbidity*

## INTRODUCTION

- Affects 2–3% of pregnancies
- 90% of cases are gestational diabetes

## CLASSIFICATION

- **Pregestational diabetes** either type I (insulin dependent) or type II (non–insulin dependent)
- **Gestational diabetes:** diabetes that develops during pregnancy (Table 20-1) [1,2]

## PRECONCEPTION COUNSELING

- Glycosylated hemoglobin (hemoglobin $A_{1C}$ <7) to assess glycemic control
- Diabetes associated with fetal anomalies if poor glucose control before pregnancy (Table 20-2)
- Anomalies reduced by improved glycemic control during embryo-genesis

## DIAGNOSIS

- All patients screened between 24 and 28 wks with 50-g nonfasting, 1-hr glucose challenge test (GCT)
- If glucose >140 mg/dL, perform 3-hr fasting glucose tolerance test (GTT)
- Two abnormal values on GTT confirm gestational diabetes
- Guidelines for interpretation of the GCT and GTT: see Table 20-3
- Early screening offered for high-risk patients (previous gestational diabetes, prior macrosomic infant, age >30, unexplained fetal demise)

### TABLE 20-1A.
### WHITE CLASSIFICATION OF DIABETES IN PREGNANCY: PART 1

| Class | Onset | Fasting glucose | 2-hr postprandial glucose | Therapy |
|-------|-------|-----------------|---------------------------|---------|
| $A_1$ | Gestational | <105 mg/dL | <120 mg/dL | Diet |
| $A_2$ | Gestational | >105 mg/dL | >120 mg/dL | Insulin |

### TABLE 20-1B.
### WHITE CLASSIFICATION OF DIABETES IN PREGNANCY: PART 2

| Class | Age at onset (yrs) | Duration (yrs) | Vascular disease | Therapy |
|-------|--------------------|-----------------|------------------|---------|
| B | >20 | <10 | None | Insulin |
| C | 10–19 | 10–19 | None | Insulin |
| D | <10 | >20 | Benign retino-pathy | Insulin |
| F | Any | Any | Nephropathy | Insulin |
| R | Any | Any | Proliferative retinopathy | Insulin |
| H | Any | Any | Heart | Insulin |

### TABLE 20-2.
### CONGENITAL ANOMALIES ASSOCIATED WITH PREGESTATIONAL DIABETES MELLITUS

| | |
|---|---|
| Caudal regression | Situs inversus |
| Renal anomalies | Heart anomaly |
| Ureter duplex | Anal/rectal atresia |
| Agenesis | Anencephaly |
| Cystic kidney | |

**TABLE 20-3.**
**ACOG CRITERIA FOR DIAGNOSIS OF**
**GESTATIONAL DIABETES**

Screening with 50-g, 1-hr glucose challenge test

Plasma glucose >140 mg/dL

Diagnosis with 100-g 3-hr glucose tolerance test

|  | National Diabetes Data Group (mg/dL) | Carpenter/Coustan Conversion (mg/dL) |
|---|---|---|
| Fasting | 105 | 95 |
| 1 hr | 190 | 180 |
| 2 hrs | 165 | 155 |
| 3 hrs | 145 | 140 |

## ANTEPARTUM MANAGEMENT
### Maternal and Fetal Complications
See Table 20-4.

### Fetal Evaluation

- U/S 18–20 wks (anomaly survey, fetal echocardiogram), 30–32 wks (abdominal circumference and estimated fetal weight)

- Antipasto monitoring (fetal activity assessment, nonstress test beginning at 32–34 wks)

### Diagnostic Evaluation

- Ophthalmologic exam (retinopathy)

- 24-hr urine for creatinine clearance and protein (nephropathy)

- TSH

- ECG (if symptomatic or long-standing diabetes)

- BP

- Weight (BMI)

- Dietary counseling (2200–2400 kcal/d for average women)

## MANAGEMENT
### Glucose Monitoring

Home glucose monitoring 7 ×/d for patients on insulin and fasting and post-breakfast in diet-controlled patients (Table 20-5).

**TABLE 20-4.**
**COMPLICATIONS OF DIABETES IN PREGNANCY**

Maternal

| | |
|---|---|
| Nephropathy | Common in pregestational diabetes |
| | Increased risk of preeclampsia |
| Retinopathy | Occurs after several years of pregestational diabetes |
| | Often deteriorates during pregnancy |
| | Evaluation by ophthalmologist every trimester |
| | Proliferative retinopathy treated with laser treatment |
| Diabetic ketoacidosis | May occur at lower glucose concentrations |
| | Treat with fluids, electrolyte replacement, IV insulin, and fetal surveillance |

Fetal complications

| | |
|---|---|
| Macrosomia (>4000–4500 g) | Increased trunk and shoulder dimensions and increased risk of shoulder dystocia |
| Fetal demise | Increased spontaneous abortion and fetal death in utero |
| | Good glycemic control decreases risk |
| Polyhydramnios | From fetal polyuria |
| Perinatal | Fetal hypoglycemia, respiratory syndrome, hyperbilirubinemia, polycythemia, hypocalcemia |

**TABLE 20-5.**
**OPTIMAL GLYCOLIC CONTROL**

| Time | Optimal glucose |
|---|---|
| Fasting | 60–90 mg/dL |
| 1 hr before meals (ac) | 60–105 mg/dL |
| Postprandial | |
| 1 hr (pc) | 130–140 mg/dL |
| 2 hr (pc) | 120 mg/dL |
| 2 a.m.–6 a.m. | 60–90 mg/dL |

Home glucose monitoring: fasting, 1 hr ac, 1 hr pc, 2 a.m.

## Diet Therapy: Initial Treatment

- 30 kcal/kg/day

- Fasting glucose levels persistently >105 mg/dL or if 2-hr postprandial values are persistently >120 mg/dL, pharmacologic treatment

## Oral Hypoglycemics

- Glyburide may be appropriate for gestational diabetes [4]: 2.5 mg daily (increased by 2.5 mg and then 5 mg every week to a max dose of 20 mg/d).

- Home glucose monitoring must be followed closely.

- Institute insulin if poor glycemic control.

## Insulin

- Hospitalize poorly controlled gestational diabetics and pregestational diabetics to tailor insulin dosage.

- Given in divided doses of regular (short acting) and neutral protamine Hagedorn insulin (intermediate acting).

- Table 20-6 outlines insulin dosing.

**TABLE 20-6.**
**INSULIN DOSAGE, ADMINISTRATION,**
**AND PHARMACOLOGY**

| | | Peak (hrs) | | | Duration (hrs) | | |
|---|---|---|---|---|---|---|---|
| Tri-mester | Insulin dosage | Reg-ular | NPH/Lente | Ultralente | Reg-ular | NPH/Lente | Ultralente |
| First | 0.7 units/kg IBW | 2–4 | 4–10 | 8–16 | 6–8 | 18–22 | 24–36 |
| Second | 0.8 units/kg IBW | 2–4 | 4–10 | 8–16 | 6–8 | 18–22 | 24–36 |
| Third | 0.9 units/kg IBW | 2–4 | 4–10 | 8–16 | 6–8 | 18–22 | 24–36 |

| Insulin administration | |
|---|---|
| a.m. (two-thirds of calculated daily dose) | 66% NPH, 33% regular |
| p.m. (one-third of calculated daily dose) | 50% regular at dinner; 50% NPH at bedtime |

IBW, ideal body weight (100 lbs for 5 ft. + 5 lbs/in. / 2.2 lb/kg).
Note: Insulin should be administered 30 min ac.

## INTRAPARTUM MANAGEMENT
### Delivery

- Patient with macrosomia or other high-risk patients may be candidates for early delivery.

- If elective delivery before 39 wks, confirm fetal lung maturity.

- Increased risk for shoulder dystocia.

- Consider elective c-section for macrosomia.

### Intrapartum Metabolic Control

- Maintain euglycemia during labor.

- Insulin drip with hourly accuchecks in labor.

- Hold scheduled insulin for patients undergoing c-section.

- Insulin given prn during c-section.

## POSTPARTUM MANAGEMENT

- Gestational diabetics have 50% chance of developing type II DM.

- 2-hr, 75-g GTT within 6 wks of delivery.

## REFERENCES

1. American College of Obstetricians and Gynecologists. Gestational diabetes. *ACOG Practice Bulletin 30.* Washington, DC: ACOG, 2001.
2. American Diabetes Association. Gestational diabetes mellitus. *Diabetes Care* 1998;21[Suppl 1]:S60–S61.
3. Miller E, Hare JW, Cloherty JP, et al. Elevated maternal hemoglobin A1C in early pregnancy and major congenital anomalies in infants of diabetic mothers. *N Engl J Med* 1981;304:1331–1334.
4. Langer O, Conway DL, Berkus MD, et al. A comparison of glyburide and insulin in women with gestational diabetes mellitus. *N Engl J Med* 2000;343:1134–1138.

# 21 Thyroid Disease

*Hypothyroidism is associated with infertility*

## HYPERTHYROIDISM

0.2% of pregnancies

### Differential Diagnosis

Exacerbations of Graves' disease are common during pregnancy and postpartum (Table 21-1).

### History

- Heat intolerance
- Tremor
- Palpitations
- Weight loss

### Physical Exam

- Thyromegaly/goiter
- Exopthalmos and pretibial myxedema (Graves' disease)
- Tachycardia

### Diagnostic Evaluation

- TSH (decreased)
- Free $T_4$ (increased)
- Thyroid-stimulating antibody for Graves' disease
- Other: CBC, LFTs

### Complications

- Preeclampsia, CHF, low-birth-weight infants
- Fetal thyrotoxicosis and goiter from transplacental passage of thyroid-stimulating antibodies
- Fetal hypothyroidism from maternal thioamides is rare

### TABLE 21-1.
### DIFFERENTIAL DIAGNOSIS OF HYPERTHYROIDISM

Graves' disease (most common)

Toxic adenoma

Thyroid neoplasm

Hyperemesis

Drugs (iodine, amiodarone)

Toxic multinodular goiter

Thyroiditis

Ingestion of thyroid hormone

Gestational trophoblastic disease

Subclinical hyperthyroidism (low TSH, normal free $T_4$)

### Management

- Thioamides: propylthiouracil (PTU) and methimazole (Tapazole, Thiamazole)
- Inhibit synthesis of $T_4$ and $T_3$ (PTU also blocks peripheral conversion of $T_4$ to $T_3$)
- Side effect of agranulocytosis in 0.2%: stop drug
- Methimazole: associated with aplasia cutis
- PTU: drug of choice
  - 100–150 mg PO q8h (starting dose)
- Increase up to 600 mg/d until response (may take 3–4 wks)
- Adrenergic blockers: symptomatic relief
- Propranolol (Inderal, Inderal LA), 40 mg PO bid (titrate to maternal pulse <100 bpm)
- Iodides: block release of stored thyroid hormone; only indicated for thyroid storm
- May result in fetal hypothyroidism
- Thyroidectomy: fail medical therapy
- Radioiodine: *absolutely contraindicated*

### THYROID STORM
### History

- Fever

- Tachycardia
- Heart failure
- Preeclampsia

**Management**

- IV hydration with monitoring of fluid balance
- PTU, 1 g
- Supersaturated potassium iodide, 5 drops q8h
- Propranolol (titrate dose to pulse <100 bpm)
- Antipyretics
- Cooling blanket
- $O_2$ by mask
- Telemetry
- Continuous fetal heart rate monitoring
- Positioning in left lateral position to maximize uterine perfusion

**HYPOTHYROIDISM**

Often results in infertility

**Differential Diagnosis**

See Table 21-2.

**History**

- Weight gain
- Lethargy
- Cold intolerance

**TABLE 21-2.**
**DIFFERENTIAL DIAGNOSIS OF HYPOTHYROIDISM**

Hashimoto's thyroiditis (most common)

Posttreatment hypothyroidism

Thyroiditis

Iodine deficiency

Drugs (iodides, lithium, thioureas)

Subclinical hypothyroidism (high TSH, normal $FT_4$)

- Muscle cramps
- Brittle nails and dry skin

**Diagnostic Evaluation**
- TSH (elevated)
- Free $T_4$ (decreased)

**Complications**
- Preeclampsia
- Placental abruption
- Low birth weight
- Stillbirths

**Management**
- Levothyroxine (Synthroid), 0.1–0.15 mg PO daily
- Patients already on Synthroid may require increased doses
- Increase dose q4wks
- TSH monitored q6–8wks

**POSTPARTUM THYROIDITIS**
- Destructive lymphocytic thyroiditis from microsomal antibodies
- Two phases: a thyrotoxic phase and a hypothyroid phase
  - Thyrotoxic phase: 4% of women, 1–4 mos postpartum
    - Symptoms from glandular destruction with hormone release
    - Thioamides ineffective
    - Beta-blockers for symptomatic treatment
  - Hypothyroid phase: 2–5% of women, 4–8 mos postpartum
    - $T_4$ replacement initiated and continued for 12–18 mos
    - Hypothyroidism permanent in 10–30%

**SUGGESTED READING**

American College of Obstetricians and Gynecologists. Thyroid disease in pregnancy. *ACOG Practice Bulletin 32*. Washington, DC: ACOG, 2001.

Masiukiewicz US, Burrow GN. Hyperthyroidism in pregnancy. *Thyroid* 1999;9:647–652.

# 22

# Human Immunodeficiency Virus

*All pregnant women should be screened for HIV*

## INTRODUCTION
In the United States, 7000 pregnancies/yr are complicated by HIV.

## PATHOPHYSIOLOGY
- HIV is a single-stranded RNA virus.
- Transmission: transplacentally, by exposure of the infant to the maternal birth canal and through breast milk [1].
- 40–80% of vertically transmitted cases occur intrapartum.

## DIAGNOSIS
- All pregnant woman are offered HIV testing.
- ELISA is the initial screening test.
- Positive ELISA is confirmed by Western blot.
- Comanage patients with an infectious disease specialist.

## ANTEPARTUM MANAGEMENT
### Diagnostic Evaluation
- Ophthalmologic, respiratory, neurologic, and pelvic exams.
- PPD, CBC, LFTs, creatinine.
- HIV viral load (q1–3mos), CD4 count (q1–4mos).
- Resistance testing is of uncertain value.

### Immunizations
- Hepatitis B vaccine if seronegative
- Pneumococcal vaccine if not vaccinated within last 5 yrs
- Influenza vaccine in the second or third trimester during influenza season

### Antiretroviral Therapy
See Table 22-1.

## TABLE 22-1.
## ANTEPARTUM ANTIRETROVIRAL THERAPY

| Clinical scenario/ question | Recommendation | |
|---|---|---|
| Clinical scenario | | |
| CD4 cell count <350 cells/mm$^3$ | Combination antiretroviral therapy | |
| Viral load >1000 copies/mL | | |
| Acute HIV syndrome | | |
| Symptoms ascribed to HIV infection | | |
| Viral load <1000 copies/mL | ZDV prophylactic therapy or combination antiretroviral therapy | |
| Common questions | | |
| Initiation of combination therapy | Antiretroviral naïve women: 10–12 wks Women already on treatment at time of pregnancy: continue throughout gestation or stop for first trimester and restart during second trimester | |
| Choosing a combination regimen | Similar to nonpregnant regimens (see below) Should include ZDV as per AIDS Clinical Trial Group 076 protocol | |
| Commonly used combination regimens | One drug from column A and one combination from column B: | |
| | Column A: | Column B: |
| | Nelfinavir (Viracept) | Didanosine (Videx) and zidovudine (Retrovir) |
| | Indinavir (Crixivan) | Lamivudine (Epivir, Epivir-HBV) and zidovudine (Retrovir) |
| | Ritonavir (Norvir) | Stavudine (Zerit) and lamivudine (Epivir, Epivir-HBV) |
| | Saquinavir (Fortovase, Invirase) | Stavudine (Zerit) and didanosine (Videx) |
| ZDV prophylactic therapy (AIDS Clinical Trial Group 076 protocol) | | |

(*continued*)

**TABLE 22-1.
(CONTINUED)**

| Clinical scenario/ question | Recommendation |
|---|---|
| Antepartum | ZDV, 100 mg 5 × daily |
| Intrapartum | ZDV, 2 mg/kg IV over 1 hr, then 1 mg/kg/hr until delivery |
| | Neonatal ZDV, 2 mg/kg q6h × 6 wks beginning 8–12 hrs after birth |
| Postpartum | Reinstitute antiviral regimen used antepartum |

ZDV, zidovudine.

## Teratology

- FDA categories and toxicity are listed in Table 22-2.

### Close monitoring for

- Nucleoside analogs (zidovudine, ddI, d4T): hepatic steatosis, lactic acidosis, myopathy (monitor electrolytes, LFTs periodically)
- Protease inhibitors: glucose intolerance

### Avoid

- Efavirenz (Sustiva): anencephaly, anophthalmia, cleft palate
- Amprenavir (Agenerase): increased propylene glycol

## Opportunistic Infections: Prophylaxis

- Pneumocystis carinii (CD4 <200/mm$^3$): TMP-SMX (Bactrim, Septra, Co-trimoxazole)
- Mycobacterium avium complex (CD4 <50/mm$^3$): azithromycin (Zithromax, Zithromax Z-Pak) weekly

## Intrapartum Management

- Immediate HIV testing if unknown sero-status.
- Avoid amniotomy and fetal scalp electrode placement if possible.

## Antiretroviral Therapy

Patients in labor should receive antiretrovirals (Table 22-3).

## Delivery

- Viral loads of >1000 copies/mL: elective c-section at 38 wks without amniocentesis offered to decrease risk of vertical transmission

**TABLE 22-2.**
**FDA CATEGORY AND TOXICITY OF ANTIRETROVIRALS**

| Drug | FDA category | Toxicity |
|---|---|---|
| Nucleoside reverse transcriptase inhibitors | | |
| Zidovudine (AZT) (Retrovir) | C | Marrow suppression |
| Zalcitabine (ddC) (Hivid) | C | Neuropathy, stomatitis |
| Didanosine (ddI) (Videx) | B | Pancreatitis, neuropathy |
| Stavudine (d4T) (Zerit) | C | Neuropathy |
| Lamivudine (3TC) (Epivir, Epivir-HBV) | C | Pancreatitis |
| Abacavir (ABC) (Ziagen) | C | Hypersensitivity |
| Nonnucleoside reverse transcriptase inhibitors | | |
| Nevirapine (Viramune) | C | Rash |
| Delavirdine (Rescriptor) | C | Rash |
| Efavirenz (Sustiva) | C | Anencephaly |
| Indinavir (Crixivan) | C | Nephrolithiasis |
| Protease inhibitors | | |
| Ritonavir (Norvir) | B | Nausea and vomiting |
| Saquinavir (Fortovase) | B | Nausea, diarrhea |
| Nelfinavir (Viracept) | B | Diarrhea |
| Amprenavir (Agenerase) | C | Increase propylene glycol |

## TABLE 22-3.
## INTRAPARTUM ANTIRETROVIRAL THERAPY

| Regimen | Maternal therapy | Neonatal therapy |
| --- | --- | --- |
| ZDV | 2 mg/kg IV bolus, then 1 mg/kg/hr until delivery | 2 mg/kg PO q6h × 6 wks |
| Nevirapine | 200 mg PO × 1 at onset of labor | 2 mg/kg PO at 48–72 hrs of life (administer as soon as possible if maternal nevirapine given <1 hr before delivery) |
| ZDV/nevirapine | ZDV, 2 mg/kg IV bolus then 1 mg/kg/hr until delivery; nevirapine, 200 mg PO × 1 at onset of labor | ZDV, 2 mg/kg PO q6h × 6 wks; nevirapine, 2 mg/kg PO at 48–72 hrs of life |
| ZDV/lamivudine | ZDV, 600 mg PO at onset of labor, then 300 mg PO q12h until delivery | ZDV 4 mg/kg PO q12 |
| | 3TC, 150 mg PO at onset of labor, then 150 mg PO q12h until delivery | Lamivudine, 2 mg/kg PO q12h for 7 d |

ZDV, zidovudine.

• Role of scheduled c-section for lower viral loads is uncertain.

### Postpartum Management

Breast feeding is contraindicated.

### SUGGESTED READING

Watts DH. Management of human immunodeficiency virus infection in pregnancy. *N Engl J Med* 2002;346:1879–1891.

Connor EM, Sperling RS, Gelber R, et al. Reduction of maternal-infant transmission of human immunodeficiency virus type I with zidovudine treatment. Pediatric AIDS Clinical Trials Group Protocol 076 Study Group. *N Engl J Med* 1994;331:1173–1180.

### REFERENCE

1. Public Health Service Task Force Perinatal HIV Guidelines Working Group. Summary of the Updated Recommendations from the Public Health Service Task Force to Reduce Perinatal Human Immunodeficiency Virus-1 Transmission in the United States. *Obstet Gynecol* 2002;99:1117–1126.

# 23 Urinary Tract Infections

*UTIs should be treated aggressively*

## ASYMPTOMATIC BACTERIURIA

- Complicates 2–9% of pregnancies.
- All patients screened at first prenatal visit with urine culture.
- Associated with low birth weight, preterm labor, symptomatic UTIs.

### Treatment

Antibiotics are described in Table 23-1; follow-up urine culture to verify cure.

## CYSTITIS
### History

- Dysuria
- Frequency
- Urgency

### Diagnostic Evaluation

UA (leukocytes, nitrites, bacteria, RBCs)

### Treatment

- Antibiotics as described in Table 23-1; follow-up urine culture to verify cure.
- Treat promptly to prevent pyelonephritis.

## PYELONEPHRITIS

- Complicates 1–2% of pregnancies.
- Right-sided pyelonephritis is most common; 25% of cases are bilateral.

### History

- Dysuria
- Nausea and vomiting

**TABLE 23-1.**
**TREATMENT REGIMENS FOR ASYMPTOMATIC**
**BACTERIURIA AND CYSTITIS**

| Drug | Dosage |
|------|--------|
| Nitrofurantoin monohydrate (Macrobid) | 100 mg PO q12h × for 3 d |
| Nitrofurantoin macrocrystals (Macrodantin) | 50–100 mg PO q6h × 3 d |
| TMP-SMX (Bactrim DS) | 160/180 mg PO q12h × 3 d |
| Cephalexin (Keflex) | 250–500 mg PO q6h × 3 d |
| If sensitivities available: | |
| Ampicillin (Omnipen, Principen, Totacillin) | 250–500 mg PO q6h × 3 d |
| Amoxicillin (Amoxil, Biomox, Polymox, Trimox, Wymox) | 250–500 mg PO q8h × 3 d |
| TMP (Proloprim, Trimpex) | 200 mg PO q12h × 3 d |
| Sulfisoxazole (Gantrisin) | 2-g load, then 1 g q6h × 3 d |

- Frequency
- Fevers and chills
- Hematuria
- Abdominal/back pain

**Physical Exam**

- Vital signs (fever, hypotension, tachycardia)
- Costovertebral angle tenderness
- Lower quadrant/flank pain

**Diagnostic Evaluation**

- UA (leukocytes, nitrites, bacteria, RBCs)
- Urine culture with sensitivities (*Escherichia coli*, *Klebsiella pneumoniae*, *Enterobacter*, and *Proteus* most common)
- Blood cultures (optional, 15% bacteremic)
- Lab: CBC, electrolytes, serum creatinine
- CXR (if pulmonary symptoms)

### Complications

- Renal dysfunction (elevated creatinine, decreased creatinine clearance)

- ARDS

- Hemolysis (secondary to endotoxin release)

- Preterm labor

### Initial Management

- Fluid hydration and electrolyte replacement

- Empiric regimens

  - Ampicillin (Omnipen, Principen, Totacillin), 2 g IV q6h and gentamicin, 2 mg/kg IV load, then 1.5 mg/kg IV q8h

  - Ceftriaxone (Rocephin), 1–2 g IV qd

  - TMP-SMX (Bactrim), 160/800 mg PO q12h

- Therapy modified based on microbial sensitivities

- Most improve in 2 d

- Therapy continued for 10–14 d with PO antibiotics

- Outpatient management considered in selected populations

- Urine culture after antibiotic treatment to verify cure

- Suppressive therapy [nitrofurantoin, (Macrobid), 50–100 mg PO qhs] for remainder of pregnancy

### Management of Nonresponders

- If no response in 48–72 hrs, rule out urinary obstruction.

- Rule out nephrolithiasis or perinephric abcess with renal U/S on single film IUP

- Renal U/S or single-film IV pyelogram

### SUGGESTED READING

Cunningham FG, Gant NF, Leveno KJ, et al., eds. *Williams obstetrics*, 21st ed. New York: McGraw-Hill, 2001.

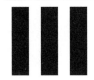

# Intrapartum Care

# 24

# Normal Labor and Delivery

*Guidelines for normal labor management*

## EVALUATION

- See Table 24-1.
- U/S if exam does not verify presentation.
- Speculum exam for nitrizine testing and ferning if loss of fluid.

## CARDINAL MOVEMENTS OF LABOR

- Mechanisms by which the fetal head navigates maternal pelvis [1].
- Engagement, descent, flexion, internal rotation, extension, external rotation, expulsion.
- See Fig. 24-1.

## STAGES OF LABOR

- First stage: uterine contractions until complete cervical dilation
  - Latent phase: onset of labor until 4-cm dilation
  - Active phase: 4-cm dilation until complete dilation
- Second stage: complete dilation until delivery of fetus
- Third stage: delivery of fetus until expulsion of placenta

### First Stage of Labor

- Assessment of fetal heart rate and contractions
- Vaginal exams q2–4h
- NPO with IV access in active phase
- Obstetric anesthesia and augmentation of labor described elsewhere

### Second Stage of Labor
#### *Normal Delivery*

- Fetal head crowns and distends the perineum.
- Delivery of the fetal head with modified Ritgen maneuver.
- Elevation of chin while pressure exerted on occiput.
- Downward traction to delivery anterior shoulder.

**TABLE 24-1.**
**EVALUATION OF MOTHER AND FETUS**

Vaginal exam

    1. Dilation: cm

    2. Effacement: cervical length

       Cm or percent (normal 4-cm cervix)

    3. Station: descent above or below ischial spines

       0 station: at ischial spines

       Divided into thirds above $(-3, -2, -1)$ and below $(+1, +2, +3)$ ischial spines

    4. Position

       Anterior, mid-position, posterior

    5. Cervical consistency

Presentation

    Fetal part that is descending in the birth canal

       1. Cephalic (vertex): head flexed with chin against chest

       2. Breech: lower half of fetal body first

Leopold's maneuvers

    1. First maneuver: What is at the fundus?

    2. Second maneuver: Where are the spine and the small parts?

    3. Third maneuver: What is the presenting part?

    4. Fourth maneuver: Where is the cephalic prominence?

Lie

    Relation of the fetal long axis to the mother

       1. Longitudinal

       2. Transverse

Position

    Fetal occiput determines for cephalic presentations. The occiput may be right or left and anterior, posterior, or transverse.

Estimated fetal weight

---

- Upward traction to deliver posterior shoulder.

- Umbilical cord doubly clamped and cut.

- Infant handed off to pediatrician or mother.

- Nuchal cord may be reduced over infant's head, doubly clamped, and cut if unreducible.

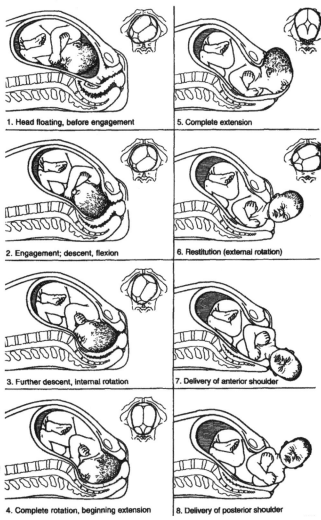

1. Head floating, before engagement
2. Engagement; descent, flexion
3. Further descent, internal rotation
4. Complete rotation, beginning extension
5. Complete extension
6. Restitution (external rotation)
7. Delivery of anterior shoulder
8. Delivery of posterior shoulder

**FIG. 24-1.**
Cardinal movements of labor. (Reprinted with permission from Cunningham FG, Gant NF, Leveno KJ, et al., eds. *Williams obstetrics*, 21st ed. New York: McGraw-Hill 2001:302.)

### Episiotomy

- Incision is made in perineum to prevent traumatic lacerations.

- Routine episiotomies are no longer performed [2].

- Indication: shoulder dystocia, breech, operative vaginal delivery, occiput posterior.

- Midline: easier to repair, heals well.

- Mediolateral: more difficult to repair, extensions to third- and fourth-degree lacerations less common.

## Third Stage of Labor
### Placental Delivery

- Signs of spontaneous separation: gush of blood, uterus rises in the abdomen, lengthening of umbilical cord

- Allow delivery without excess traction

- Excess traction may cause cord avulsion, uterine inversion

- Placenta delivers within 30 mins

- No separation: manual extraction or curettage

### Lacerations: Classification

- First degree: involve only the vaginal mucosa

- Second degree: involve the underlying fascia or muscles but not the anal sphincter

- Third degree: involve the anal sphincter

- Fourth degree: extend through rectal mucosa

### Repair

- See Fig. 24-2.

- 2-0 or 3-0 chromic or Vicryl.

- Vaginal mucosa closed in running fashion to hymenal ring.

- Distal to hymenal ring, the submucosa is closed in running fashion.

- Mucosa then closed with interrupted stitches or with subcuticular stitch.

- Anal sphincter must be repaired for third- and fourth-degree lacerations.

## FETAL ASSESSMENT
### Apgar Scores

- See Table 24-2.

- Determine need and success of neonatal resuscitation.

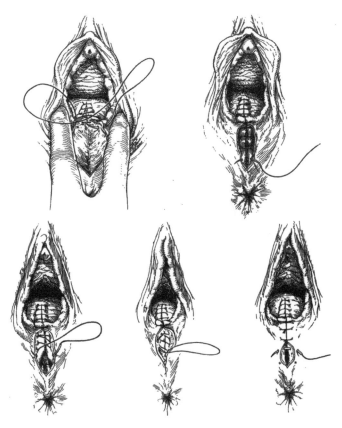

**FIG. 24-2.**
Repair of an episiotomy or laceration. (Reprinted with permission from Cunningham FG, Gant NF, Leveno KJ, et al., eds. *Williams obstetrics*, 21st ed. New York: McGraw-Hill 2001:327.)

- Not useful to assess hypoxia or neurologic damage.

## Umbilical Artery Acid-Base Analysis

- See Table 24-3.

- Assessing fetal hypoxia.

- Segment of umbilical cord is doubly clamped at delivery.

- 1–2 mL of blood aspirated from umbilical artery into syringe previously flushed with heparin.

**TABLE 24-2.**
**APGAR SCORES**

|  | 0 | 1 | 2 |
|---|---|---|---|
| Heart rate | Absent | <100 bpm | >100 bpm |
| Respirations | Absent | Weak, hypoventilation | Good, crying |
| Muscle tone | Limp | Some flexion | Active motion |
| Reflex irritability | No response | Grimace | Vigorous cry, withdrawal |
| Color | Blue or pale | Body pink; extremities blue | Completely pink |

**TABLE 24-3.**
**UMBILICAL ARTERY ACID-BASE ANALYSIS**

|  | pH | Partial pressure of $CO_2$ | Bicarbonate |
|---|---|---|---|
| Respiratory acidosis | <7.20 | High | Normal |
| Metabolic acidosis | <7.20 | Normal | High |
| Mixed acidosis | <7.20 | High | Low |

- Acidosis: pH <7.20 (severe if <7.00).

- Then assess partial pressure of $CO_2$ (mean, around 49–50) and bicarbonate (mean, around 22–23).

## SUGGESTED READING

American College of Obstetricians and Gynecologists. Use and abuse of the Apgar score. *ACOG Committee Opinion 174*. Washington, DC: ACOG, 1996.

## REFERENCES

1. Cunningham FG, Gant NF, Leveno KJ, et al., eds. *Williams obstetrics*, 21st ed. New York: McGraw-Hill, 2001.
2. Argentine Episiotomy Trial Collaborative Group. Routine versus selective episiotomy: A randomized controlled trial. *Lancet* 1993;342:1515.

# 25 Intrapartum Fetal Monitoring

*Intrapartum monitoring is an integral part of modern obstetrics*

## FETAL HEART RATE

- External fetal monitor (EFM) or internal fetal scalp electrode (FSE)
- FSE more accurate assessment but requires rupture of membranes [1]

### Indications

- No difference in intrapartum death rates between continuous monitoring and intermittent auscultation [2]
- ACOG guidelines:
  - Active labor: auscultation or EFM strip evaluation q15mins
  - Second stage: auscultation or EFM strip evaluation q5mins

### Baseline

- Normal: 120–160 bpm
- Bradycardia: baseline <120 bpm for at least 15 mins
  - Etiology: prolonged decelerations, fetal acidemia, congenital heart block, maternal hypothermia
- Tachycardia: baseline >160 bpm
  - Etiology: chorioamnionitis, maternal fever, cardiac arrhythmias, sympathomimetic drugs

### Variability

Normal fetal heart rate exhibits beat-to-beat changes secondary to autonomic nervous activity.

#### Short-Term Variability

- Changes in fetal heart rate from 1 beat to the next
- Can only be measured with FSE

#### Long-Term Variability

- Changes in fetal heart rate over 1 min
- Decreased or absent long-term variability is most reliable sign of fetal acidemia, compromise

- Other causes of decreased long-term variability: analgesics, $MgSO_4$

## Accelerations

- Increases in fetal heart rate above baseline
- Reactive: two 15-sec accelerations of at least 15 bpm in 20 mins
- Sign of fetal well-being

## Decelerations

Decreases in fetal heart rate below baseline

## Variable Deceleration

- Result of umbilical cord compression
- Occur any time in relation to contraction
- Abrupt onset and return to baseline
- Prolonged, severe variable decelerations with loss of variability are sign of impending fetal acidosis
- Management: place FSE, give $O_2$, change maternal position, discontinue oxytocin, begin amnioinfusion
- Prolonged deceleration: terbutaline (Brethaire, Brethine, Bricanyl) (0.125 mg IV or SC)

## Early Decelerations

- See Fig. 25-1.
- Result of fetal head compression.
- Begin with a contraction and end shortly after contraction.
- Symmetric shape.
- Common in second stage of labor.
- Management: usually none required.

## Late Decelerations

- See Fig. 25-2.
- Result of uteroplacental insufficiency.
- Begin after the peak of a contraction.
- Return to baseline after the contraction.
- Smooth, rarely drop >40 bpm below baseline.
- Management: FSE, give $O_2$, change maternal position.

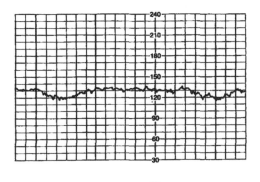

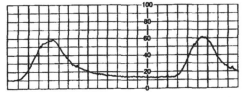

**FIG. 25-1.**
Early deceleration. (Reprinted from Cunningham, MacDonald PC, Gant NF, et al., eds. *Williams obstetrics*, 20th ed. Philadelphia: Appleton & Lange, 1997:357, with permission.)

- Repetitive late decelerations are an ominous sign: fetal scalp sampling or delivery required.

### Sinusoidal Heart Rate

- See Fig. 25-3.
- Regular oscillations around baseline.
- Etiology: fetal anemia, analgesics, severe acidosis.
- Diagnostic criteria:
  - Baseline: 120–160 bpm
  - Loss of short term variability
  - Amplitude of 5–15 bpm above and below baseline
  - 3–5 cycles/min

### UTERINE CONTRACTIONS

- Measured by external tocodynamometer or intrauterine pressure catheter (IUPC)

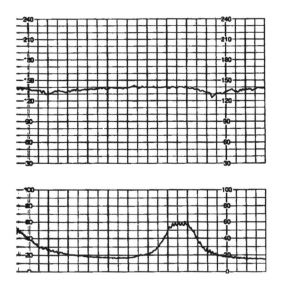

**FIG. 25-2.**
Late deceleration. (Reprinted from Cunningham FB, MacDonald PC, Gant NF, et al., eds. *Williams obstetrics*, 20th ed. Philadelphia: Appleton & Lange, 1997:359, with permission.)

- Intensity can only be quantitated by IUPC
- Contraction strength calculated in Montevideo units
  - Calculate units above baseline for all contractions in a 10-min period

## AMNIOINFUSION

- Infusion of normal saline into the uterine cavity through IUPC
- Applications: variable decelerations, meconium *only really useful to dilute meconium.*
- Protocol: 600-cc bolus, then 180 cc/hr of normal saline

## FETAL SCALP SAMPLING

- Determine fetal pH.
- If acidemia noted, operative delivery indicated.
- If pH is normal, labor may continue.

### Procedure

- Amnioscope placed in vaginal vault, head visualized

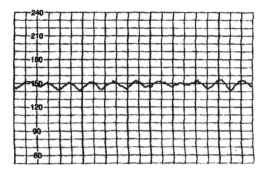

**FIG. 25-3.**
Sinusoidal heart rate. (Reprinted with permission from Cunningham FG, Gant NF, Leveno KJ, et al., eds. *Williams obstetrics*, 21st ed. New York: McGraw-Hill, 2001:340.)

- Area on scalp dried with a swab, coated with silicone gel
- Small puncture made on fetal scalp
- Blood collected into capillary tube and pH immediately measured

**Management**

See Table 25-1.

**FETAL PULSE OXIMETRY**

- Continuous monitoring of fetal $O_2$ saturation by transcervical catheter against fetal cheek
- Risk of fetal acidosis low if fetal $O_2$ saturation remains >30%
- If fetal $O_2$ saturation <30% for >10 mins, incidence of fetal acidosis increases [3]

**TABLE 25-1.**
**FETAL SCALP PH**

| pH | Management |
| --- | --- |
| >7.25 | Observe (continue labor) |
| 7.20–7.25 | Repeat sample in 30 mins |
| <7.20 | C-section |

## OTHER TECHNIQUES

Vibroacoustic stimulation or fetal scalp stimulation performed for decreased variability

## REFERENCES

1. American College of Obstetricians and Gynecologists. Fetal heart rate patterns: monitoring, interpretation, and management. *ACOG Technical Bulletin 207*. Washington, DC: ACOG, 1995.
2. Leveno KJ, Cunningham FG, Nelson S, et al. A prospective comparison of selective and universal electronic fetal monitoring in 34,995 pregnancies. *N Engl J Med* 1986;315:615–619.
3. Garite TJ, Dildy GA, McNamara H, et al. A multicenter controlled trial of fetal pulse oximetry in the intrapartum management of non-reassuring fetal heart rate patterns. *Am J Obstet Gynecol* 2000;183:1049–1058.

# 26 Induction and Augmentation of Labor

*A variety of methods exists for labor induction*

## FETAL LUNG MATURITY

- Document fetal lung maturity (FLM) for elective delivery before 39 wks (Table 26-1).

- Amniotic fluid obtained by amniocentesis.

- Cascade system used when sequential tests of FLM are performed [1].

  - If any test is positive, no further testing necessary.

## BISHOP SCORE
Predicts likelihood of successful induction of labor (Table 26-2) [2,3]

## CERVICAL RIPENING
Cervical ripening agents used if irregular/absent contractions (Table 26-3)

### Prostaglandins
### *Prostaglandin $E_2$ (Dinoprostone)*

- Gel or vaginal insert

- Side effects: uterine hyperstimulation, vomiting, and diarrhea

- Bronchoconstriction not a side effect

### *Prostaglandin $E_1$ (Misoprostol, Cytotec)*

- Not FDA approved for labor indication but commonly used

- Administered orally or vaginally

- Uterine hyperstimulation more common than with prostaglandin $E_2$ misoprostol

- Contraindicated in patients with prior c-section (risk of increased uterine rupture)

### Mechanical Methods
### *Laminaria japonicum*

- Osmotic dilators placed in cervix

- May be associated with increased risk of postpartum infection

## TABLE 26-1.
## FETAL LUNG MATURITY

| Test | Positive fetal lung maturity | Comment |
|------|------------------------------|---------|
| Lecithin-sphingo-myelin ratio | >2.0 | Blood and meconium interfere |
| Phosphatidylglycerol | Positive | Not affected by blood, meconium |
| | | Late appearance in amniotic fluid |
| Foam stability index | >47–48 | Blood and meconium interfere |
| TDx–fetal lung maturity | >50 | Often first-line test |

## TABLE 26-2.
## BISHOP SCORE

| Score | Dilation (cm) | Efface-ment (%) | Station | Cervical consistency | Position of cervix |
|-------|---------------|-----------------|---------|----------------------|--------------------|
| 0 | Closed | 0–30 | –3 | Firm | Posterior |
| 1 | 1–2 | 40–50 | –2 | Medium | Mid-position |
| 2 | 3–4 | 60–70 | –1, 0 | Soft | Anterior |
| 3 | 5–6 | 80 | +1, +2 | — | — |

| Score | Chance of success (%) |
|-------|------------------------|
| 0–4 | 50–60 |
| 5–9 | 80–90 |

### Foley Balloon

- 24–30 French Foley balloon placed into cervix for mechanical dilation

### Amniotomy

- Shortens duration of labor
- Umbilical cord prolapse risk if fetal head not well applied to cervix

### Membrane Stripping

- Sweeping a finger between uterine wall and amniotic membrane
- Possible increased rate of chorioamnionitis

## TABLE 26-3.
## METHODS OF INDUCTION OF LABOR

| Method | Procedure | Comments |
|---|---|---|
| Prostaglandins | | |
| Prostaglandin E$_2$ | | |
| Gel (Prepidil) | 2.5-mL syringe apply q6h | Max, 3 doses |
| Vaginal insert (Cervidil) | Apply vaginally q12h | Contraindicated if prior c-section |
| Prostaglandin E$_1$ (Cytotec) | 25–50 µg q4–6h vaginally | |
| Mechanical methods | | |
| Laminaria japonicum | Inserted into cervical os | |
| Foley balloon | Inserted into cervical os | Falls out when cervix dilates |
| Amniotomy | | |
| Membrane stripping | | |

| Oxytocin | Starting dose (mU/min) | Incremental increase (mU/min) | Dosage interval (mins) |
|---|---|---|---|
| Low-dose regimens | 0.5–1 | 1 | 30–40 |
| | 1–2 | 6 | 15 |
| High-dose regimens | 6 | 2 | 15 |
| | 6 | 6 or 3 or 1 | 20–40 |

## OXYTOCIN

- IV oxytocin used to induce labor if cervix favorable or augment labor for patients already in labor
- Many regimens
- Complications: uterine hyperstimulation, water intoxication

## REFERENCES

1. American College of Obstetricians and Gynecologists. Assessment of fetal lung maturity. *ACOG Educational Bulletin 230.* Washington, DC: ACOG, 1996.

2. American College of Obstetricians and Gynecologists. Induction of labor. *ACOG Practice Bulletin 10*. Washington, DC: ACOG, 1999.
3. Bishop EH. Pelvic scoring for elective induction. *Obstet Gynecol* 1964;24:266–268.

# 27

# Dystocia

*Dystocia is a major cause of neonatal morbidity*

## INTRODUCTION

- **Dystocia:** difficult labor
- **Etiology:** abnormalities in uterine contractility (powers), the fetus (passenger), or maternal pelvis (passage)

## CLASSIFICATION

### Normal Labor

First stage divided into latent and active phases

- **Latent phase:** until cervix is 3–4 cm dilated; irregular contractions
- **Active phase:** 4 cm until delivery of infant; contractions more frequent

### Abnormal Labor

- **Protraction disorders:** slower than normal progress (Table 27-1).
- **Arrest disorders:** cessation of progress (see Table 27-1).
- Arrest of the first stage not diagnosed until active phase entered and uterine contractions have been adequate (>200 Montevideo units) for a minimum of 2 hrs.
- Arrest disorders: many patients benefit from up to 6 hrs of adequate contractions if fetal well-being present.
- Friedman curve (graphic display of normal labor): See Fig. 27-1.

## POWERS

- During active phase 3–5 contractions (minimum of 200–240 Montevideo units) usually present in 10-min period
- Management: amniotomy or oxytocin

### Passenger

- Fetal causes of dystocia: macrosomia, malpresentation, fetal anomalies
- Estimate fetal weight by Leopold's maneuver or U/S
- Macrosomia may require c-section
- Malpresentation discussed in Chap. 28, Malpresentation

**TABLE 27-1.**
**CRITERIA FOR DIAGNOSIS OF PROTRACTION AND ARREST DISORDERS**

|  | Nulligravidas | Multigravidas |
|---|---|---|
| Prolonged latent phase | >20 hrs | >14 hrs |
| Protraction disorders |  |  |
| Dilation | <1.2 cm/hr | <1.5 cm/hr |
| Descent | <1.0 cm/hr | <2.0 cm/hr |
| Arrest disorders |  |  |
| Dilation | >2 hrs | >2 hrs |
| Descent | >1 hr | >1 hr |
| Second stage | >2 hrs (3 hrs with epidural anesthesia) | >1 hr (2 hrs with epidural anesthesia) |

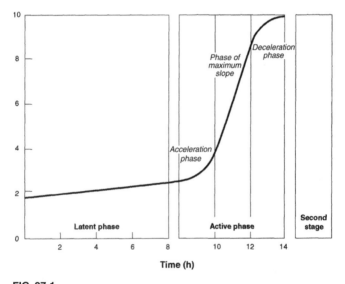

**FIG. 27-1.**
Friedman curve of normal labor. (Reprinted with permission from Friedman EA. *Labor: evaluation and management*, 2nd ed. East Norwalk, CT: Appleton-Century-Croft, 1978.)

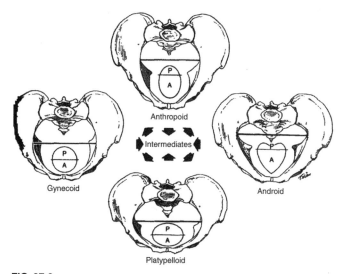

**FIG. 27-2.**
Caldwell-Moloy classification of female pelvic types. (Reprinted with permission from Cunningham FG, Gant NF, Leveno KJ, et al., eds: *Williams obstetrics*, 21st ed. New York: McGraw-Hill, 2001:57.)

- **Asynclitism:** sagittal suture is deviated anteriorly or posteriorly
- **Abnormalities of position:** manual rotation or forceps delivery

## PASSAGE

- Perform clinical pelvimetry on all patients.
- Inadequate bony pelvis often requires c-section.
- Caldwell-Moloy classification (Fig. 27-2).
- Gynecoid pelvis most common.

### Clinical Pelvimetry
#### *Pelvic Inlet*

- Pelvic inlet (obstetric conjugate) cannot be measured manually.
- Estimated by measuring diagonal conjugate from sacral promontory to the lower border of symphysis pubis.
- Normal diagonal conjugate >11.5 cm.

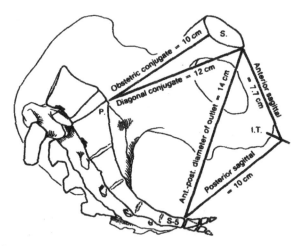

**FIG. 27-3.**
Measurement of the pelvic inlet. (Reprinted with permission from Cunningham FG, Gant NF, Leveno KJ, et al., eds. *Williams obstetrics*, 21st ed. New York: McGraw-Hill, 2001:55.)

### *Midpelvis*

- Estimated by the biischial diameter between ischial spines

- Normally >10.5 cm

### *Pelvic Outlet*

- Estimated by measuring the distance between ischial tuberosities (Fig. 27-3).

- Place a closed fist between ischial tuberosities on the perineum.

- Normal ischial tuberosity distance >8 cm.

### SELECTED READING

American College of Obstetricians and Gynecologists. Dystocia and the augmentation of labor. *ACOG Technical Bulletin 218*. Washington, DC: ACOG, 1995.

Cunningham FG, Gant NF, Leveno KJ, et al., eds. *Williams obstetrics*, 21st ed. New York: McGraw-Hill, 2001.

Friedman EA. *Labor: evaluation and management*, 2nd ed. East Norwalk, CT: Appleton-Century-Croft, 1978.

# 28 Malpresentation

*Shoulder dystocia is an obstetrics emergency*

## EVALUATION

### Presentation

- Portion of the fetus that presents in the birth canal
- Cephalic presentation: head presents
  - **Vertex (occiput):** head flexed against fetal chest
  - **Face:** fetal neck extended
  - **Brow:** fetal neck partially extended
- **Breech presentation:** fetal buttocks or lower extremity presents

### Position

- Orientation of presenting part to maternal right or left (Figs. 28-1 and 28-2)
- Vertex presentation: occiput defines fetal position
  - Posterior fontanelle of fetus identifies fetal position relative to maternal pelvis
  - Occiput may be right or left and anterior, posterior, or transverse
- Face presentation: mentum defines fetal position
  - Mentum anterior, posterior, or transverse

### Risk Factors for Malpresentation

- Fetal anomalies
- Placenta previa
- Polyhydramnios
- Macrosomia
- Uterine malformations
- Multiparity
- Pelvic neoplasms
- Prematurity
- Multiple gestation

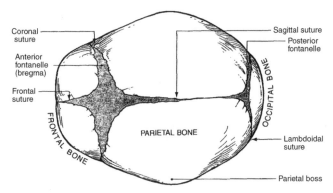

**FIG. 28-1.**
Fetal skull with anterior and posterior fontanels demonstrated.
(Reprinted with permission from Gabbe SG, Niebyl JR, Simpson JL, eds.
*Obstetrics: normal and problem pregnancies*, 4th ed. New York:
Churchill Livingstone, 2002:358.)

## BREECH PRESENTATION

- 3% of pregnancies at delivery
- Maternal and fetal morbidity increased [1]

### Classification

- See Fig. 28-3.
- **Frank:** both hips flexed, both knees extended.
- **Complete:** both hips flexed, one or both knees flexed.
- **Incomplete:** one or both hips extended.

### Management

C-section, vaginal breech delivery, or external version (if not in labor)

#### *External Cephalic Version [2]*

- Attempted after 36 wks before active labor
- Fetus manually turned to vertex presentation
- Success rate, 50–70%
- Tocolytics and epidural anesthesia may increase success
- External fetal monitoring and access for emergency c-section should be available
- Complications: abruption, fetal death, return to nonvertex presentation

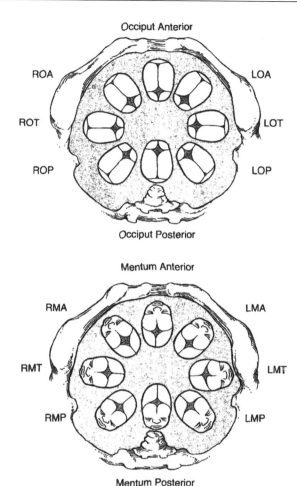

Occiput Anterior

ROA    LOA

ROT    LOT

ROP    LOP

Occiput Posterior

Mentum Anterior

RMA    LMA

RMT    LMT

RMP    LMP

Mentum Posterior

**FIG. 28-2.**
Fetal position. (Reprinted with permission from Gabbe SG, Niebyl JR, Simpson JL, eds. *Obstetrics: normal and problem pregnancies*, 4th ed. New York: Churchill Livingstone, 2002.)

## Vaginal Breech Delivery

- Attempted in highly selected patients.

- Mother must be informed of increased risk of complications [3].

- Selection criteria: see Table 28-1.

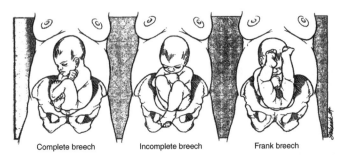

Complete breech    Incomplete breech    Frank breech

**FIG. 28-3.**
Breech presentations. (Reprinted with permission from Gabbe SG, Niebyl JR, Simpson JL, eds. *Obstetrics: normal and problem pregnancies*, 4th ed. New York: Churchill Livingstone 2002:482.)

*Procedure*

- Infant allowed to deliver spontaneously to umbilicus
- Both legs then swept across midline and freed
- Downward traction exerted until scapula is visualized
- Infant then rotated and both arms swept across chest and freed
- Head delivered
- Piper forceps may assist delivery of head
- Mauriceau-Smellie-Veit: fetus rests on palm of attendant's hand while fingers of attendant are applied to fetal maxilla to aid head flexion

### FACE PRESENTATION

- 1 in 600 deliveries.
- C-section if persistent mentum posterior.

### TABLE 28-1.
### CRITERIA FOR VAGINAL BREECH DELIVERY

| | |
|---|---|
| Frank breech | Adequate pelvis |
| Fetal weight <4000 g | Fetal head not hyperextended |
| Anesthesia available | Capability of emergent c-section |
| No IUGR | Availability of physician with vaginal breech delivery experience |
| Gestational age >36–37 wks | |

- Mentum anterior presentations may undergo vaginal delivery.
- Manual or forceps rotations avoided.
- C-section if obstructed labor.

## BROW PRESENTATION

- 1 in 1500 deliveries
- Often convert to vertex or face presentation
- Brow presentation may deliver vaginally
- If labor obstructed, c-section

## TRANSVERSE LIE

- 1 in 360 deliveries
- Often shoulder presentation
- C-section or external cephalic version

## COMPOUND PRESENTATION

- Extremity is prolapsed next to the presenting part
- Do not manipulate prolapsed extremity
- C-section if labor obstructed or umbilical cord prolapse

## OCCIPUT POSTERIOR POSITION

- Usually rotate to occiput anterior
- If dystocia develops: forceps rotation, forceps-assisted vaginal delivery, vacuum-assisted delivery, or manual rotation

## OCCIPUT TRANSVERSE POSITION

- Often rotate to occiput anterior or occiput posterior positions
- May attempt forceps rotation with increased risk for fetal morbidity
- C-section usually indicated

## SHOULDER DYSTOCIA

- Fetal shoulder becomes impaction after delivery of fetal head
- 1–4% of pregnancies
- Neonatal morbidity: clavicular and brachial plexus injuries
- First step in management: prevention and preparedness
- >50% of patients with shoulder dystocia have no risk factors and fetal weights <4000 g

## TABLE 28-2.
## MANAGEMENT OF SHOULDER DYSTOCIA

| | |
|---|---|
| 1. Call for help | 6. Rubin's maneuver |
| 2. McRobert's maneuver | 7. Delivery of posterior arm |
| 3. Suprapubic pressure | 8. Clavicular fracture |
| 4. Episiotomy | 9. Repeat steps 2, 3, 5, and 6 |
| 5. Wood's screw maneuver | |

### Risk Factors

- Macrosomia
- DM
- Obesity
- Multiparity
- Prolonged second stage of labor

### Management

- See Table 28-2.
- Suprapubic pressure: affects delivery of anterior shoulder.
- **McRobert's maneuver:** flexing mother's legs against her chest may free impacted fetal shoulder.
- **Wood's screw maneuver:** rotation of posterior shoulder 180 degrees to aid release of anterior shoulder.
- **Rubin's maneuver:** compressing either of neonate's shoulders toward chest.
- Delivery of posterior arm: usually frees anterior shoulder.
- Clavicular fracture.
- **Zavanelli maneuver:** replacing neonatal head into maternal pelvis with emergent c-section.

### REFERENCES

1. American College of Obstetricians and Gynecologists. Mode of term singleton breech delivery. *ACOG Committee Opinion 265.* Washington, DC: ACOG, 2001.
2. American College of Obstetricians and Gynecologists. External cephalic version. *ACOG Practice Bulletin 13.* Washington, DC: ACOG, 2000.

3. Hannah ME, Hannah WJ, Hewson SA, et al. Planned c-section versus planned vaginal birth for breech presentation at term: a randomized multicentre trial. *Lancet* 2000;356:1375–1383.

## SUGGESTED READING

Gabbe SG, Niebyl JR, Simpson JL, eds. *Obstetrics: normal and problem pregnancies*, 4th ed. New York: Churchill Livingstone, 2002.

Cunningham FG, Gant NF, Leveno KJ, et al., eds. *Williams obstetrics*, 21st ed. New York: McGraw-Hill, 2001.

# 29 Intrapartum Complications

*Common intrapartum complications*

## GROUP B STREPTOCOCCUS (GBBS OR *STREPTOCOCCUS AGALACTIAE*)

### Microbiology

- Colonizes maternal genitourinary and GI tracts
- 10–30% of pregnant women colonized with GBBS
- Vertical transmission at delivery results in serious neonatal morbidity

### Pathology

- Maternal infections: chorioamnionitis, urinary tract and wound infections
- Neonatal infections:
  - Early-onset disease: onset <7 d from delivery
    - Sepsis with respiratory failure
    - 25% mortality
    - Antibiotic treatment of the newborn ineffective
  - Late-onset disease: onset >7 d after birth
    - Meningitis
    - Vertical transmission (50%) or nosocomial spread (50%)

### Prophylaxis

- Universal screening of all patients now recommended (Fig. 29-1) [1–3].
  - Patients with positive cultures treated during labor with IV antibiotics.
  - All patients should have GBBS culture of vagina and rectum at 35–37 wks.
- Guidelines for patients with preterm labor: see Fig. 29-2.
- Antibiotic selection for prophylaxis: see Table 29-1.

# GROUP B STREPTOCOCCUS (GBBS OR *Streptococcus agalactiae*)

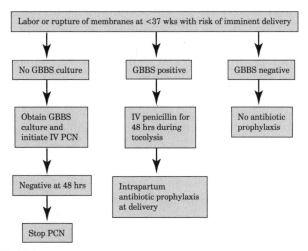

GBBS culture (vaginal and rectal) at 35–37 wks on all pregnant patients (except those with GBBS bacteriuria in current pregnancy or a previous infant with GBBS disease)

Intrapartum prophylaxis
- Positive GBBS culture during current pregnancy (unless planned cesarean section without labor)
- Previous infant with invasive GBBS disease
- GBBS bacteriuria during current pregnancy
- Unknown GBBS status with:
  - Delivery at <37 wks
  - ROM >18 hrs
  - Intrapartum fever (>38°C)

NO intrapartum prophylaxis
- Negative GBBS culture during current pregnancy REGARDLESS of other intrapartum risk factors
- Planned cesarean section without labor or rupture of membranes
- Previous pregnancy with positive GBBS culture

**FIG. 29-1.**
Recommendations for GBBS prophylaxis. (Adapted from Schrag S, Gorwitz R, Fultz-Butts K, et al. Prevention of perinatal group B streptococcal disease. Revised guidelines from CDC. *MMWR Recomm Rep* 2002;51[RR-11]:1–22.)

Labor or rupture of membranes at <37 wks with risk of imminent delivery

No GBBS culture

GBBS positive

GBBS negative

Obtain GBBS culture and initiate IV PCN

IV penicillin for 48 hrs during tocolysis

No antibiotic prophylaxis

Negative at 48 hrs

Intrapartum antibiotic prophylaxis at delivery

Stop PCN

**FIG. 29-2.**
Recommendations for GBBS prophylaxis for patients with threatened preterm labor. (Adapted from Schrag S, Gorwitz R, Fultz-Butts K, et al. Prevention of perinatal group B streptococcal disease. Revised guidelines from CDC. *MMWR Recomm Rep* 2002;51[RR-11]:1–22.)

**TABLE 29-1.**
**ANTIBIOTIC PROPHYLAXIS FOR GBBS**

Preferred: Penicillin G, 5 million U, then 2.5 million U IV q4h

Alternate: Ampicillin (Omnipen, Principen, Totacillin), 2 g, then 1 g IV q4h

Nonanaphylactoid penicillin allergy: Cefazolin (Ancef), 1 g IV q8h

Anaphylactoid penicillin allergy:

　GBBS sensitivities at 34–36 wks

　　Clindamycin (Cleocin Oral, Cleocin T), 900 mg IV q8h

　　Erythromycin (E-Mycin, E.E.S., Ery-Tab, Eryc, EryPed, Ilosone), 500 mg IV q8h

　Clindamycin- and erythromycin-resistant GBBS

　　Vancomycin (Lyphocin, Vancocin HCl, Vancocin HCl Pulvules, Van-coled, Vancomycin HCl), 1 g IV q12h

## CHORIOAMNIONITIS

- Infection of the fetal membranes
- Complications: preterm labor, PROM, dysfunctional labor, neonatal sepsis

### Microbiology

- Ascending infection
- Usually polymicrobial: GBBS, gram-negative rods, and anaerobes

### Risk Factors

- Prolonged rupture of membranes
- Multiple vaginal exams
- Prolonged labor
- GBBS colonization

### Physical Exam

- Vital signs (fever, maternal and fetal tachycardia)
- Uterine tenderness
- Malodorous amniotic discharge
- Nonreassuring fetal tracing
- Dysfunctional labor
- Leukocytosis

## Diagnosis

- Based on clinical findings
- Amniocentesis if preterm labor and PROM
- Amniotic fluid: culture, Gram's stain, leukocyte count, and glucose level

## Management

- Antibiotic treatment and delivery
- Augmentation of labor for term and preterm patients
- C-section if dystocia develops
- Antibiotic regimen: ampicillin, 1–2 g IV q6h with gentamycin, 2 mg/kg loading dose, then 1.5 mg/kg q8h
- Increased risk of postpartum endomyometritis

## MECONIUM

- Passage of meconium occurs in 10–15% of pregnancies.
- Normal process after the maturation of fetal GI tract.
- In some fetuses, meconium passage may signal fetal hypoxia and gasping.

## Pathology

- Neonatal morbidity from fetal aspiration of meconium-stained amniotic fluid
- Mechanical obstruction of bronchial tree and chemical pneumonitis

## Diagnosis

- Identification of green-stained amniotic fluid at time of membrane rupture

## Treatment

- Prophylactic amnioinfusion is often used
- At delivery, suction infant's nose and mouth with DeLee suction at perineum
- Neonatal intubation with suction to level of vocal cords

## CORD PROLAPSE

- Obstetric emergency
- Umbilical cord protrudes through cervix below fetal presenting part
- Cord occlusion and fetal hypoxia result

- Management: fetal presenting part should be elevated during vaginal exam and emergent c-section

## REFERENCES

1. American College of Obstetricians and Gynecologists. Prevention of early-onset group B streptococcal disease in newborns. *ACOG Committee Opinion 279*. Washington, DC: ACOG, 2002.
2. Schrag S, Gorwitz R, Fultz-Butts K, et al. Prevention of perinatal group B streptococcal disease. Revised guidelines from CDC. *MMWR Recomm Rep* 2002;51(RR-11):1–22.
3. Schrag SJ, Zell ER, Lynfield R, et al. A population-based comparison of strategies to prevent early-onset group B streptococcal disease in neonates. *N Engl J Med* 2002;347(4):233–239.
4. Hager DW, Schuchat A, Gibbs R, et al. Prevention of perinatal group B streptococcal infection: current controversies. *Obstet Gynecol* 2000;96:141–145.

# 30

# Operative Obstetrics

*Forceps and vacuum*

## FORCEPS DELIVERY
### Safety

- Elective forceps safe

- Increased incidence of perineal trauma, maternal hematomas

### Classification

- ACOG classification shown in Table 30-1.

- High forceps not included.

### Indications

- Maternal indications: cardiopulmonary disease, neurologic disease, infection, maternal exhaustion, prolonged second stage of labor

- Fetal-fetal distress, nonreassurring fetal status

### Preparation

Table 30-2 lists prerequisites for forceps application.

### Application

- See Fig. 30-1.

- Right hand placed between fetal head and left side of maternal pelvis.

- Left blade then introduced with the left hand into the left side of the maternal pelvis.

- Left blade gently guided into place.

- Left hand then placed between right maternal pelvic wall and the fetal head.

- Right blade then introduced with right hand into right side of maternal pelvis.

### Traction

- Placement verified

- Gentle horizontal traction applied until head bulges at perineum

## TABLE 30-1.
## CLASSIFICATION OF FORCEPS DELIVERIES

Outlet forceps

    1. Scalp visible at introitus without labial separation

2. Fetal skull has reached the pelvic floor

3. Sagittal suture is in anteroposterior diameter or right or left occiput anterior or posterior position

4. Fetal head is at or on perineum

5. Rotation not >45 degrees

Low forceps

1. Leading point of fetal skull is at station >+2 cm and not on the pelvic floor

2. Rotation is ≤45 degrees (left or right occiput anterior to occiput anterior, or left or right occiput posterior to occiput posterior)

3. Rotation is >45 degrees

Midforceps

1. Station is above +2 cm but head is engaged

Reprinted from the American College of Obstetricians and Gynecologists. *Operative Vaginal Delivery (Practice Bulletin No. 17).* Washington, DC: ACOG, June 2000, with permission.

- Handles then gently elevated until infant's head delivers
- Forceps then disengaged

### VACUUM EXTRACTION

Indications and preparation similar to forceps

## TABLE 30-2.
## PREREQUISITES FOR FORCEPS DELIVERY

1. Head must be engaged

2. Vertex presentation

3. Position must be known

4. Cervix completely dilated

5. Membranes ruptured

6. Adequate pelvis

7. Adequate anesthesia

8. Bladder emptied

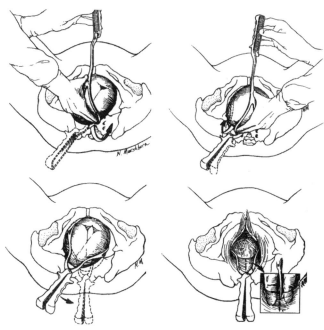

**FIG. 30-1.**
Forceps application. (Reprinted with permission from Cunningham FG, Gant NF, Leveno KJ, et al., eds. *Williams obstetrics*, 21st ed. New York: McGraw-Hill, 2001;493–494.)

## Safety

Complications: cephalohematoma (14–16%), subgaleal hematomas, intracranial hemorrhage, neonatal hyperbilirubinemia, retinal hemorrhage

## Application

- Cup is placed over the sagittal suture anterior to posterior fontanelle
- Placement verified
- Suction then applied and traction affected with maternal expulsive efforts
- Dislodgement of cup is common cause of failure
- Dislodgement minimized by gently anchoring cup against fetal head with operator's hand during traction

## REFERENCES

1. American College of Obstetricians and Gynecologists. Operative vaginal delivery. *ACOG Practice Bulletin 17*. Washington, DC: ACOG, 2000.
2. Cunningham FG, Gant NF, Leveno KJ, et al., eds. *Williams obstetrics*, 21st ed. New York: McGraw-Hill, 2001.

# 31 Obstetric Anesthesia

*Regional anesthesia is now commonly used during labor*

## PHYSIOLOGY

- First stage: pain from uterine contractions and cervical dilation
  - Visceral afferent fibers to T-10 through L-1
- Second stage: pain from distention of the genital tract
  - Pudendal nerve (S-2 through S-4)

## SYSTEMIC ANALGESIA

- IV analgesics commonly administered during early labor
- Complications: hypotension, nausea, and vomiting
- Neonatal neurologic and respiratory depression occur if delivery occurs before opioid affects are relieved
- Common agents
  - Butorphanol (Stadol), 1–2 mg IV or IM q3–4h
  - Nalbuphine (Nubain), 10 mg IV or IM q3–6h
  - Meperidine (Demerol), 25–50 mg IV q3–4h often with
  - Promethazine (Phenergan), 25 mg IV q3–4h
  - Fentanyl sublimase, 50–100 µg q1h
- Neonatal respiratory depression: naloxone (0.1 mg/kg IV) can be given

## EPIDURAL ANESTHESIA

- Catheter into the epidural space at the L2–L3, L3–L4, or L4–L5.
- Local anesthetic (bupivacaine, lidocaine, 2-chloroprocaine) administered by continuous infusion.
- Opioid (fentanyl or sufentanil) may also be administered.
- Appropriate for vaginal delivery and c-section.
- See Table 31-1.

### Contraindications

- Coagulopathy
- Thrombocytopenia

**TABLE 31-1.**
**COUNSELING PATIENTS ON EPIDURAL**

Epidural anesthesia is generally safe.

The risk of paralysis is very, very small.

The effects on labor are debated.

Side effects include hypotension, headaches, and urinary retention.

- Infection at the site of placement
- Hypovolemia
- No available trained personnel
- Increased ICP

## Complications
### Hypotension

- Bolus of 500–1000 cc of normal saline may be administered before epidural placement
- Management: bolus of normal saline, ephedrine (5–10 mg IV)
- Fetal decelerations often occur during hypotension

### Systemic Toxicity

- CNS symptoms: dizziness, metallic taste, tinnitus, convulsions
- Cardiovascular symptoms follow: hypotension, arrhythmias
- Test dose of epinephrine given before dosing the epidural
- Management: supportive care

### Total Spinal Blockade

- Secondary to injection into subarachnoid space
- Paralysis and respiratory failure may occur
- Management: supportive

### Postpuncture Headache

- Secondary to leakage of CSF at site of spinal puncture
- Develops postpartum, exacerbated by position changes
- Management: bed rest, caffeine, blood patch

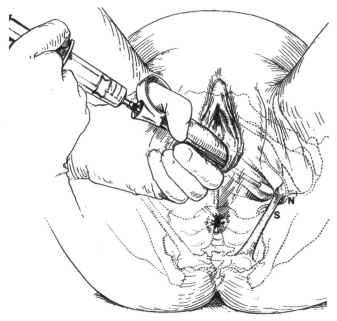

**FIG. 31-1.**
Pudendal block. N, pudendal nerve; S, sacrospinous ligament. (Reprinted with permission from Cunningham FG, Gant NF, Leveno KJ, et al., eds. *Williams obstetrics*, 21st ed. New York: McGraw-Hill 2001:371.)

### *Other: Epidural Abscess, Hematoma, Meningitis*

• Urinary retention common.

• Effect of epidural on the progress of labor is debated.

### SPINAL ANALGESIA

• Injection of opioids into the spinal (intrathecal) space.

• Common for c-section, may be used for vaginal delivery.

• Contraindications and complications similar to epidural anesthesia.

### PUDENDAL BLOCK

• May provide adequate analgesia for vaginal delivery (Fig. 31-1).

• 7–10 mL of 1% lidocaine injected into each pudendal nerve.

• Needle tip is placed below the ischial spine.

- Aspirate before injection to ensure the pudendal artery has not been entered.

## SUGGESTED READING

American College of Obstetricians and Gynecologists. *Obstetric analgesia and anesthesia. ACOG Practice Bulletin 36.* Washington, DC: ACOG, 2002.

Cunningham FG, Gant NF, Leveno KJ, et al., eds. *Williams obstetrics,* 21st ed. New York: McGraw-Hill, 2001.

# IV

## Postpartum

# 32

# Postpartum Infection

*Postpartum infections are a significant source of maternal morbidity*

## INTRODUCTION

Postpartum fever: temperature elevation to $\geq 38.0^{\circ}$C ($100.4^{\circ}$F) on any 2 of the first 10 d postpartum exclusive of the first 24 hrs

## DIFFERENTIAL DIAGNOSIS

See Table 32-1.

## DIAGNOSTIC EVALUATION

See Table 32-2.

## ENDOMYOMETRITIS

Puerperal infection of the uterine cavity

### Risk Factors

- C-section
- Prolonged rupture of membranes
- Multiple vaginal exams
- Prolonged labor
- Preexisting infections
- Low socioeconomic status
- Anemia

### Microbiology

- Polymicrobial infection (anaerobes, gram-negatives, gram-positive cocci, *Chlamydia*) by vaginal flora
- Bacteremia in 10–20%

### Diagnosis

- Based on clinical exam
- Fever, abdominal pain, fundal tenderness, foul lochia

### Management

- Regimens

**TABLE 32-1.**
**DIFFERENTIAL DIAGNOSIS OF POSTPARTUM FEVER**

| Complication | System | Comments |
|---|---|---|
| Womb | Uterine: endomyo-metritis; septic pelvic thrombophlebitis | See below |
| Wound | Wound: infection; breakdown | Risk factors: diabetes, obesity, steroids, infection, immunodeficiency, poor surgical technique |
| | | Diagnosis: wound erythema, tenderness, induration, pus |
| | | Treatment: open and débride wound, verify fascia intact, wound cleaning and débridement bid–tid, antibiotics if infection |
| Wind | Pulmonary: atelectasis; aspiration; pneumonia | Atelectasis: incentive spirometry |
| | | Pneumonia: antibiotics |
| | | Pneumonia may occur later (>24 hrs) after atelectasis resolved |
| Wean | Breast: engorgement; mastitis | Engorgement: ice packs, breast support, fever usually low grade |
| | | Avoidance of suckling will enhance breast involution |
| | | Mastitis: *S. aureus*; continue breast feeding; dicloxacillin, 500 mg qid |
| Water | Renal: cystitis; pyelonephritis | Diagnosis: urine culture |
| | | Treatment: antibiotics |
| Wonder drugs | Meds | Discontinue drugs |
| Walking | DVT | Diagnosis: lower extremity Doppler |
| | | Treatment: heparin or low-molecular-weight heparin followed by coumadin |

- Ampicillin, 2 g IV q6h; clindamycin (Cleocin), 900 mg IV q8h; gentamycin, 2-mg/kg loading dose, then 1.5 mg/kg q8h (peak and trough with third dose)

- Ampicillin, 2 g IV q6h; metronidazole (Flagyl), 500 mg IV q6h; gentamycin, 2-mg/kg loading dose, then 1.5 mg/kg q8h (peak and trough with third dose)

## TABLE 32-2.
## DIAGNOSTIC EVALUATION OF POSTPARTUM FEVEᴚ

Physical exam

Breast exam

CBC

U/A and urine culture

Blood cultures (optional)

CXR (pulmonary symptoms)

Lower extremity Doppler (deep venous thrombosis symptoms)

Breast milk culture (breast symptoms)

CT scan (persistent fever to rule out abscess, septic pelvic thrombophlebitis)

- Pipercillin-tazobactam (Zosyn), 3.375 g IV q4–6h
- Antibiotics continued until afebrile 48 hrs
- No oral regimen needed after parenteral therapy unless abscess, bacteremia, or unusual organism

### Prevention

Prophylactic antibiotics (cefazolin, cefotetan) for c-section, PROM

### SEPTIC PELVIC THROMBOPHLEBITIS

- Bacterial seeding of venous endothelial layer stimulating thrombosis
- Signs and symptoms
  - Similar to endomyometritis
  - Acute thrombosis with localized symptoms and adnexal mass
- Symptoms improve with antibiotics, but patients continue to have high spiking fevers (enigmatic fevers)
- Diagnosis: clinical presentation, CT, or MRI
- Treatment: continued antibiotics, heparin

### SUGGESTED READING

Brown CE, Stettler RW, Twickler D, et al. Puerperal septic pelvic thrombophlebitis: incidence and response to heparin therapy. *Am J Obstet Gynecol* 1999;181(1):143–148.

Cunningham FG, Gant NF, Leveno KJ, et al., eds. *Williams obstetrics*, 21st ed. New York: McGraw-Hill, 2001.

# 33 Postpartum Psychiatric Disorders

*All new mothers should be monitored for postpartum depression and psychosis*

## INTRODUCTION
Risk factors for postpartum psychiatric disorders

- Pregnancy complications
- Pregnancy loss
- Poor social support
- Low self-esteem
- Marital problems
- Unwanted pregnancy
- History of postpartum depression
- Young age
- Personal or family history of depression

## POSTPARTUM BLUES
- Affects 50% of pregnancies.
- Develops 3–6 d after delivery.
- Insomnia, poor concentration, irritability, labile affect, tearfulness.
- Suicidal ideation or delusions should trigger assessment for psychosis.
- *Treatment*: personal support, adequate rest, reassurance.
- Symptoms mild and resolve by 2 wks postpartum.

## POSTPARTUM DEPRESSION
- Affects 8–15% of pregnancies.
- Develops within 2–3 mos of delivery.
- Diagnostic criteria same as for major depressive episode.
- *Treatment*: antidepressants.
  - Fluoxetine (Prozac), 20–40 mg qam PO
  - Paroxetine (Paxil), 20–50 mg qam PO

**TABLE 33-1.**
**DIAGNOSTIC CRITERIA FOR MAJOR**
**DEPRESSIVE EPISODE**

Five of the following symptoms for a 2-wk period. One symptom must be depressed mood or loss of interest or pleasure every day.

1. Depressed mood most of day

2. Diminished interest in all or most activities

3. Significant weight loss or gain

4. Insomnia or hypersomnia

5. Psychomotor agitation or retardation

6. Fatigue or energy loss

7. Guilt or feelings of worthlessness

8. Diminished concentration

9. Recurrent suicidal ideations without a plan

• Symptoms impair social or occupational functioning

• Symptoms are not due to medical condition or substance abuse

• Symptoms are not within 2 mos of loss of a loved one

- • Sertraline (Zoloft), 50–200 mg qd PO
- • Citalopram (Celexa), 20 mg qd PO
- • Fluvoxaminze (Luvox), 50 mg qhs PO (usually to 100–300 mg divided bid)
- • Most patients improve over 6 mos (although risk for recurrence is high).
- • Monitored for suicide infanticide.
- • Psychiatric consultation: atypical or severe symptoms.
- • See Table 33-1.

## POSTPARTUM PSYCHOSIS

- • Affects 1–4 mothers/1000 births.
- • Develops 10–14 d postpartum.
- • Inability to discern reality, disorientation, psychosis.
- • Women with underlying psychiatric disorder tend to relapse postpartum.
- • *Treatment*: psychiatric consultation, antipsychotics.

- Infants removed to prevent infanticide.

- Many develop relapsing psychotic episodes.

## SUGGESTED READING

Cunningham FG, Gant NF, Leveno KJ, et al., eds. *Williams obstetrics*, 21st ed. New York: McGraw-Hill, 2001.

# 34 Postpartum Hemorrhage

*Postpartum hemorrhage must be recognized and treated promptly*

## INTRODUCTION

- >500 cc blood loss in the first 24 hrs after delivery or 10% change in Hct between admission and delivery

- **Early postpartum hemorrhage:** occurs in the first 24 hrs after delivery

- **Late postpartum hemorrhage:** occurs 24 hrs–6 wks postpartum

## DIFFERENTIAL DIAGNOSIS

See Table 34-1.   *4 T's*

### Uterine Atony   *TONE*

- Uterus fails to contract after delivery

- Risk factors

  - Uterine overdistention (hydramnios, multiple gestation, macrosomia)

  - Rapid or prolonged labor

  - Uterine relaxing agents (magnesium, halogenated anesthetics, terbutaline)

  - High parity

  - Oxytocin

  - Chorioamnionitis

- *Initial treatment*: bimanual massage, oxytocin, other uterotonics (Table 34-2)

### Retained Placenta   *TISSUE*

- May occur alone or with placenta accreta

- Risk factors for placenta accreta: previous c-section, curettage, placenta previa, high parity

- Management: manual extraction or uterine curettage

- Placenta accreta may require hysterectomy

**TABLE 34-1.**
**DIFFERENTIAL DIAGNOSIS OF**
**POSTPARTUM HEMORRHAGE**

| Early postpartum hemorrhage | Late postpartum hemorrhage |
| --- | --- |
| Uterine atony  *TONE* | Infection |
| Retained placenta  *TISSUE* | Coagulopathy |
| Genital tract laceration  *TRAUMA.* | Retained products |
| Uterine rupture | |
| Uterine inversion | |
| Placenta accreta | |
| Coagulopathy  *THROMBIN.* | |

## Genital Tract Lacerations

- Risk factors: forceps, vacuum extraction, macrosomia, precipitous labor
- *Treatment*: suture

## Uterine Inversion

- Often secondary to excess traction on umbilical cord

**TABLE 34-2.**
**UTEROTONICS**

| | Dose | Route | Contraindications |
| --- | --- | --- | --- |
| Oxytocin | 10–40 U in 1000 cc normal saline | IV (IM, IU) Infusion | None |
| Methylergono-vine (Meth-ergine) | 0.2 mg | IM (IU) q2–4h | HTN |
| Prostaglandin F 2 α (Hemabate) | 0.25 mg | IM (IU) q15–90mins | Active cardiac, pulmonary, renal, or liver diseases |
| Misoprostol | 200–800 µg | — | Rectal |
| Dinoprostone (PGE2) | 20 mg | PR q2h | Hypotension |

Adapted from Dildy GA, Clark SL. Postpartum hemorrhage. *Contemp Obstet Gynecol* 1993;38:21–29.

- Risk factors: macrosomia, fundal placentation, oxytocin, primigravidity

- *Treatment*: manual replacement of uterus; if unsuccessful a halogenated anesthetic given followed by uterine replacement

### Uterine Rupture

- Risk factors: previous c-section, trauma, uterine surgery

- *Treatment*: surgical repair or hysterectomy

### Acquired or Hereditary Coagulopathies

- Platelet count and fibrinogen are best indicators

## PHYSICAL EXAM

- Uterine palpation

- Inspection of the genital tract for lacerations

- Inspection of the placenta

- Manual exploration of the uterine cavity

## DIAGNOSTIC EVALUATION

- Vital signs

- Monitor volume status

- CBC

- PT, PTT, fibrinogen if DIC suspected

- Type and cross for 2–4 U of packed RBCs

## MANAGEMENT

- General measures
  - IV access (1 or 2 16- to 18-gauge catheters)
  - Bladder catheterization (assists uterine contractility)
  - Fluid resuscitation with crystalloid
  - Transfusion (packed RBCs if needed)
  - Supplemental $O_2$
- Treatment of specific etiologies described above
- Maneuvers for refractory bleeding
  - Uterine packing
  - Uterine artery ligation [1]
  - Hypogastric artery ligation (value questioned)

- Hysterectomy
- Uterine artery embolization
- Military antishock trousers

## SUGGESTED READING

Dildy GA, Clark SL. Postpartum hemorrhage. *Contemp Obstet Gynecol* 1993;38:21–29.

## REFERENCE

1. O'Leary JL, O'Leary JA. Uterine artery ligation for control of post-cesarean section hemorrhage. *Obstet Gynecol* 1974;43:849–853.

# V

## Ultrasound and Genetics

# 35

# Ultrasound

*Practice is key to becoming proficient in ultrasound*

## FIRST TRIMESTER ULTRASOUND

See Table 35-1.

### Intrauterine Gestational Sac

- Identified by 5 wks with transvaginal U/S (TVS); 6 wks with transabdominal U/S (TAS)

- Mean sac diameter (MSD):

  MSD = (Length + Width + Height) / 3

  $$\text{Menstrual age} = \frac{\text{MSD} + 30}{7}$$

- MSD increases by 1 mm/day

### Crown-Rump Length

- Accurate within 5 d between wks 8 and 13

- Measured from rhombencephalon to rump

- Yolk sac not included in measurement

- Crown rump lengths listed in appendix

### Nonviable Intrauterine Gestation

- Criteria

  - MSD >25 mm (TAS) without visible embryo (blighted ovum)

  - MSD >18 mm (TVS) without visible embryo (blighted ovum)

  - Embryo >5 mm with no visible cardiac activity (nonviable embryo)

### Second Trimester Ultrasound

- Value of routine U/S questioned [1,2]

### Gestational Age

- Accuracy

  - First trimester U/S: accurate within 1 wk

  - Second trimester U/S: accurate to within 2 wks

  - Third trimester U/S: accurate to within 3 wks

**TABLE 35-1.**
**LANDMARKS OF FIRST TRIMESTER U/S**

| Landmark | Menstrual wks | hCG |
| --- | --- | --- |
| Gestational sac | 5 wks (TVS)/6 wks (TAS) | 1000–2000 (TVS) |
| | | 6500 (TAS) |
| Yolk sac | 5.5 wks (TVS)/7 wks (TAS) | 7200 |
| | MSD 8 mm (TVS) | |
| | MSD 20 mm (TAS) | |
| Embryo | 6 wks (TVS)/7 wks (TAS) | |
| | MSD 5–12 mm | |
| Fetal cardiac activity | 6 wks (TVS)/7 wks (TAS) | 10,000 |
| | MSD 12–18 mm (TVS) | |
| | MSD 25 mm (TAS) | |

MSD, mean sac diameter; TAS, transabdominal U/S; TVS, transvaginal U/S.

## Biometry

- Parameters to calculate estimated fetal weight (Fig. 35-1)
  - **Biparietal diameter:** measured at level of thalamus, falx, cavum septum pellucidum, and choroid plexus in the atria of lateral ventricles
    - Calipers placed on outer border of one cranium, inner border opposite cranium
  - **Head circumference:** measured at the level of the biparietal diameter
  - **Femur length:** measured along diaphyseal shaft excluding femoral epiphysis
  - **Abdominal circumference:** measured at level of the portal vein, stomach, and spine
- Nomograms of estimated fetal weights in appendix

## AMNIOTIC FLUID
### Amniotic Fluid Index (AFI)

Divide abdomen into four quadrants through the umbilicus; measure largest pocket of amniotic fluid in each.

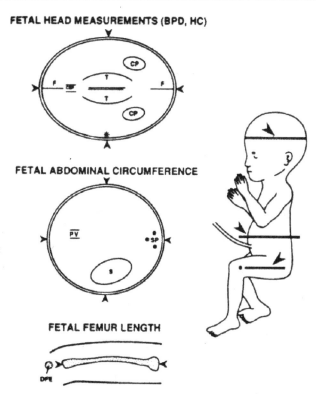

**FIG. 35-1.**
U/S planes for estimated fetal weight. BPD, biparietal diameter; CP, choroid plexus; DPE, distal epiphysis; F, falx; HC, head circumference; PV, portal vein; S, stomach; SP, spine; T, thalami. (Reprinted from Callen PW, ed: *Ultrasonography in obstetrics and gynecology*, 4th ed. Philadelphia, WB Saunders, 2000, with permission.)

**TABLE 35-2.**
**COMPONENTS OF THE BIOPHYSICAL PROFILE**

| Component | Score 2 | Score 0 |
|---|---|---|
| Fetal movement | ≥3 or more movements | <3 movements |
| Fetal tone | 1 flexion/extension motion | No flexion/extension motions |
| Fetal breathing | 30 secs breathing | <30 secs breathing |
| Amniotic fluid | 1-cm pocket | No 1-cm pocket |
| Nonstress test | Reactive | Nonreactive |

### Deepest Vertical Pocket (DVP)

- Maximum depth of any amnioticfluid pocket
- Oligohydramnios: AFI <5 cm; DVP <1–2 cm
- Polyhydramnios: AFI >20 cm; DVP >8 cm

### Biophysical Profile

- Measurement of fetal well-being (Table 35-2)
- Allotted maximum of 90 mins

### SUGGESTED READING

Callen PW, ed. *Ultrasonography in obstetrics and gynecology*, 4th ed. Philadelphia: WB Saunders, 2000.

### REFERENCES

1. Crane JP, LeFevere ML, Winborn RC, et al. A randomized trial of prenatal ultrasonographic screening: impact on the detection, management, and outcome of anomalous fetuses. *Am J Obstet Gynecol* 1994;171:392.
2. Ewigman BG, Crane JP, Frigoletto FD, et al. Effect of prenatal ultrasound screening on perinatal outcome. *N Engl J Med* 1993;329:821.

# 36

# Genetics

*Genetic counseling and testing are important parts of prenatal care*

## CHROMOSOMAL ANOMALIES
### Introduction

- 1 in 150 livebirths
- 50% of stillbirths have chromosomal anomalies
- Turner syndrome (45XO) most common
- Frequency increases with maternal age
- **Aneuploidy:** number of chromosomes is < or >46

### Trisomy 21 (Down Syndrome)

- Etiology: maternal nondisjunction (95%), translocations, or mosaicism (5%).
- Diagnosis: fetal karyotype, U/S.
- Management: counseling, offer termination.
- Recurrence rate in subsequent pregnancies: 1–2%.
- See Fig. 36-1.

### Trisomy 18 (Edward's Syndrome) and Trisomy 13 (Patau Syndrome)

- Severe mental retardation
- Stillbirths and neonatal deaths common
- Diagnosis: karyotype, U/S
- See Fig. 36-2.

### 45XO (Turner Syndrome)

- Not associated with maternal age.
- Usually secondary to absent paternal sex chromosome.
- Mosaicisms common.
- Spontaneous abortion common.
- Intelligence usually normal, some patients may reproduce.

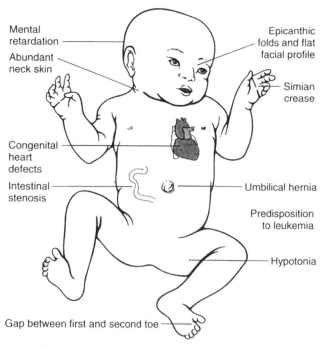

**FIG. 36-1.**
Features of trisomy 21. (Reprinted from Cotran RS, Kumar V, Collins T, et al. *Robbin's pathologic basis of disease*, 6th ed. Philadelphia: WB Saunders, 1999:172, with permission.)

- See Fig. 36-3.

## SINGLE GENE DEFECTS
### Fragile X Syndrome

- Most common cause of mental retardation in U.S.

- 1 in 1200 males and 1 in 2500 females

- Genetics: caused by expansion of a trinucleotide sequence

- Variable number of CGG nucleotide sequences are found on the X chromosome

- 50–200 copies of the repeat sequence: asymptomatic

- >200 repeats: clinical effects

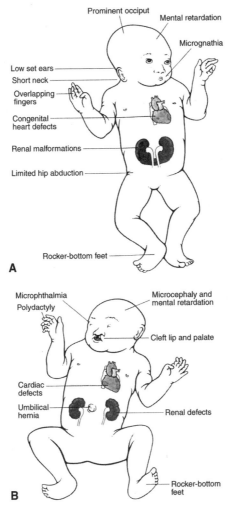

**FIG. 36-2.**
Features of trisomy 18 (A) and trisomy 13 (B). (Reprinted from Cotran RS, Kumar V, Collins T, et al. *Robbin's pathologic basis of disease*, 6th ed. Philadelphia: WB Saunders, 1999:172, with permission.)

- Degree of mental retardation more severe in males

- Clinical features: mental retardation, macroorchidism, narrow facies

- Diagnosis: PCR, Southern blot

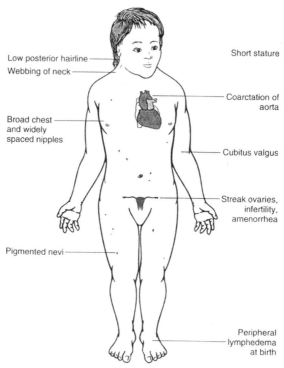

**FIG. 36-3.**
Features of Turner syndrome. (Reprinted from Cotran RS, Kumar V, Collins T, et al. *Robbin's pathologic basis of disease*, 6th ed. Philadelphia: WB Saunders, 1999:175, with permission.)

- Offer genetic counseling: parents of mentally retarded or autistic children, family history of fragile X syndrome or mental retardation

- Genetic testing of parents offered after genetic counseling

## Cystic Fibrosis

- 1 in 3300 white children [1]

- Genetics: autosomal recessive

- Many mutations possible

- 75% of affected individuals have mutations at position 508

- Clinical features

  - Meconium ileus

## TABLE 36-1.
## COMMON MENDELIAN DISORDERS

| Autosomal dominant | Autosomal recessive |
| --- | --- |
| von Willebrand's disease | Sickle cell anemia |
| Neurofibromatosis | Hemochromatosis |
| Marfan syndrome | Cystic fibrosis |
| Adult polycystic kidney disease | Wilson's disease |
| Huntington's disease | Beta thalassemia |
| Tuberous sclerosis | Phenylketonuria |
| Osteogenesis imperfecta tarda | Homocystinuria |
| Familial hypercholesterolemia | Alpha$_1$-antitrypsin deficiency |
| X-linked disorders | |
|    Hemophilia A and B | |
|    Fragile X syndrome | |
|    Testicular feminization | |
|    Color blindness | |
|    Fabry's disease | |

- COPD
- Pancreatic exocrine insufficiency
- Cirrhosis
- Life expectancy: variable (from childhood to 50–60s)
- Offer carrier screening to
  - Parents with a family history of cystic fibrosis
  - Reproductive partners of individuals with cystic fibrosis
  - Couples in whom one or both partners are white and are planning a pregnancy or seeking prenatal care
- When both partners are carriers prenatal diagnosis offered

## MULTIFACTORIAL DEFECTS

- Do not follow mendelian patterns of inheritance (Table 36-1).
- Common multifactorial disorders: neural tube defects, congenital heart disease, cleft lip cleft palate.
- Recurrence risk: 1–5%.

## SUGGESTED READING

Cotran RS, Kumar V, Collins T. *Robbin's pathologic basis of disease*, 6th ed. Philadelphia: WB Saunders, 1999.

## REFERENCE

1. American College of Obstetricians and Gynecologists. *Preconception and prenatal carrier screening for cystic fibrosis. Clinical and laboratory guidelines*. Washington, DC: ACOG, 2001.

# 37

# Prenatal Diagnosis

*Multiple marker screening should be offered to all women*

## INTRODUCTION

- Chromosomal anomalies occur in 50% of early pregnancy losses.
- 0.65% of infants are born with a chromosomal anomaly.

## SECOND TRIMESTER SCREENING
### Maternal Serum Screening

- Employs serum AFP, hCG, and unconjugated estriol to screen for Down syndrome and neural tube defects (Table 37-1)

### Interpretation

- Performed between 15 and 20 wks' gestation
- Accurate dating is essential

### Neural Tube Defects

- 85% are detected by serum screening
- Evaluation
  - U/S to examine fetal spine and cerebrum if maternal serum AFP is above 2.0–2.5 multiples of the median
  - Amniocentesis if no etiology for elevated AFP on U/S
  - Amniotic fluid AFP and acetylcholinesterase elevated
    - Karyotype may also be performed
    - Other etiologies of elevated maternal serum AFP in Table 37-2

### Trisomy 21

- Calculation of risk is made based on level of three analytes and a woman's age-related risk of Down syndrome.
- If age-related risk is greater than that of a 35-yr-old woman, the screen is considered positive.
  - U/S and amniocentesis are offered for positive screen (Table 37-3).

### TABLE 37-1.
### ANALYTES USED IN MATERNAL SERUM SCREENING

|  | Maternal serum AFP | Estriol | hCG |
| --- | --- | --- | --- |
| Trisomy 21 | Decreased | Decreased | Increased |
| Trisomy 18 | Decreased | Decreased | Decreased |
| Neural tube defect | Increased | Normal | Normal |

- Second trimester serum screening detects 60% of Down syndrome fetuses in women aged <35 and 75% of affected fetuses in women aged >35 [1].

### FIRST TRIMESTER SCREENING
#### Maternal Serum Screening

- Under investigation
- Commonly used analytes: hCG, pregnancy-associated plasma protein A (PAPP-A)
- Trisomy 21 associated with elevated hCG and decreased PAPP-A [2]

#### Nuchal Lucency Measurement

- Obtained by measuring the fetal neck.
- Increased nuchal lucency associated with Down syndrome (sensitivity 27–89%).

### TABLE 37-2.
### CONDITIONS WITH ELEVATED AFP

| | |
| --- | --- |
| Multiple gestation | Ventral wall defects |
| Fetal demise | Omphalocele |
| Fetal-maternal hemorrhage | Gastroschisis |
| Placental abnormalities | Bilateral renal agenesis |
| Uterine anomalies | Congenital skin disorders |
| Maternal dermoid cyst | Epidermolysis bullosa |
| Maternal hepatoma | Aplasia cutis |
| Neural tube defects | Sacrococcygeal teratoma |
| Congenital nephrosis | Triploidy |

**TABLE 37-3.**
**AGE-BASED RISK OF DOWN SYNDROME AND OTHER ANEUPLOIDIES**

| Maternal age | Midtrimester | | Term liveborn | |
|---|---|---|---|---|
| | Trisomy 21 | All aneuploidies | Trisomy 21 | All aneuploidies |
| 33 | 1/417 | 1/208 | 1/625 | 1/345 |
| 34 | 1/333 | 1/152 | 1/500 | 1/278 |
| 35 | 1/250 | 1/132 | 1/384 | 1/204 |
| 36 | 1/192 | 1/105 | 1/303 | 1/167 |
| 37 | 1/149 | 1/83 | 1/227 | 1/130 |
| 38 | 1/115 | 1/65 | 1/175 | 1/103 |
| 39 | 1/89 | 1/53 | 1/137 | 1/81 |
| 40 | 1/69 | 1/40 | 1/106 | 1/63 |
| 41 | 1/53 | 1/31 | 1/81 | 1/50 |
| 42 | 1/41 | 1/25 | 1/64 | 1/39 |
| 43 | 1/31 | 1/19 | 1/50 | 1/30 |
| 44 | 1/25 | 1/15 | 1/38 | 1/24 |
| 45 | 1/19 | 1/12 | 1/30 | 1/19 |

Copyright 1983, American Medical Association. Hook EB, Cross PK, Schreinemachers DM. Chromosomal abnormality rates at amniocentesis and in live-born infants. *JAMA* 1983;249:2034–2038.

## PRENATAL DIAGNOSIS

- Used to obtain fetal karyotype
- Indications in Table 37-4

### Amniocentesis

- Performed at 15–20 wks
- Fetal cells in the amniotic fluid are analyzed
- Complications: fetal loss (0.5%), mild vaginal spotting, fluid leakage, chorioamnionitis
- Early amniocentesis (11–13 wks) associated with pregnancy loss rate of 2.5%

### Chorionic Villus Sampling (CVS)

- Performed at 10–12 wks' gestation.

## TABLE 37-4.
## INDICATIONS FOR PRENATAL DIAGNOSIS

Maternal age >35 at the time of birth

Maternal serum screen risk equal to that of a 35-yr-old

Previous pregnancy complicated by autosomal trisomy

Major structural defect on U/S

Previous pregnancy complicated by sex chromosome aneuploidy

Mother or father with chromosome translocation

Mother or father is a carrier of chromosome inversion

Parental aneuploidy

- Chorionic villi are aspirated and analyzed.
- Performed transabdominally or transcervically.
- Complications: fetal loss rate (1–2%).
- Early CVS (7–9 wks) associated with limb reduction and oromandibular defects.

### Percutaneous Umbilical Blood Sampling (PUBS, Cordocentesis)

- Direct sampling of the fetal blood and rapid karyotype analysis.
- Fetal loss: < 2%.

### SUGGESTED READING

Callen PW, ed. *Ultrasonography in obstetrics and gynecology*, 4th ed. Philadelphia: WB Saunders, 2000.

### REFERENCES

1. Haddow JE, Palomaki GE, Knight GJ, et al. Prenatal screening for Down's syndrome with use of maternal serum markers. *N Engl J Med* 1992;327:588–593.
2. Haddow JE, Palomaki GE, Knight GJ, et al. Screening of maternal serum for fetal Down's syndrome in the first trimester. *N Engl J Med* 1998;338:955–961.

# 38 Fetal Anomalies

*Know the features of common fetal anomalies*

## GASTROINTESTINAL ANOMALIES
### Abdominal Wall Defects

- Omphalocele and gastroschisis (Table 38-1)
- Management: routine follow-up U/S, route of delivery dictated by obstetric indications, surgical correction after birth

### Duodenal Atresia

- Incidence: 1 in 10,000 births.
- Diagnosis: "double bubble" sign on U/S (dilated stomach and duodenum), polyhydramnios.
- 30% of fetuses have trisomy 21.

## NERVOUS SYSTEM DEFECTS
### Neural Tube Defects (NTDs)

- Failure of neural tube to close between days 26 and 28 of gestation
- Folate supplementation decreases risk of NTDs
- **Anencephaly:** fatal anomaly with absence of cranium
  - Polyhydramnios, malpresentation often accompanies defect
- **Spina bifida:** opening in vertebral column
  - **Meningocele:** meningeal sac herniates
  - **Meningomyelocele:** herniation of meninges and spinal cord
  - **Meningoencephalocele:** herniation of meninges, spinal cord and brain
  - U/S findings: "banana sign" (exaggerated cerebellar curve), "lemon sign" (scalloping of frontal bones), cerebellar herniation (Arnold-Chiari malformation)

## Choroid Plexus Cysts (CPCs)

- Incidence: 2–4% of pregnancies.
- Most are normal variants.
- Aneuploidy found in 2% of fetuses.

**TABLE 38-1.**
**FEATURES OF OMPHALOCELE AND GASTROSCHISIS**

|  | Omphalocele | Gastroschisis |
|---|---|---|
| Incidence | 2.5/10,000 | 1.75–2.5/10,000 |
| Herniation | Through umbilicus | Right of umbilicus |
| Peritoneal covering | Yes | No |
| Associated anomalies | Common | Rare |
| Survival | 50% | 80–90% |

- If other anomalies are visualized on U/S, amniocentesis offered to rule out trisomy 18 and trisomy 21.

## CARDIOVASCULAR DEFECTS
### Structural Defects

- Most common: atrioventricular septal defects (17%), ventricular septal defects (15.5%), tetralogy of Fallot (VSD, right ventricular obstruction, overriding aorta and right ventricular hypertrophy)

### Arrhythmias

- Isolated premature atrial contractions (PACs) are most common (80%). PACs are transient and require no treatment.

- Tachyarrhythmias may result in nonimmune hydrops.

## GENITOURINARY ANOMALIES

- Fetal renal pelvic dilation >4 mm followed with serial sonography.

- Most cases of mild pyelectasis are normal variants.

- Etiology of urinary obstruction: ureteropelvic junction obstruction, distal ureteral obstruction, collection system duplication and posterior urethral valves.

## THORACIC ANOMALIES

Fetal pulmonary mass: pulmonary sequestration, cystic adenomatoid malformation, and congenital diaphragmatic hernia

### Congenital Diaphragmatic Hernia

- Incidence: 1–4.5 in 10,000 infants

- Incomplete fusion of diaphragm with herniation of abdominal contents into thorax

- U/S: visualization of loops of bowel in the thorax, small abdominal circumference, mediastinal shift

- 50% have other anomalies

## FACIAL ANOMALIES

- Cleft lip and cleft palate common
- Inheritance: multifactorial (recurrence in subsequent births for the mother: 4%)

## SUGGESTED READING

Callen PW, ed. *Ultrasonography in obstetrics and gynecology*, 4th ed. Philadelphia: WB Saunders, 2000.

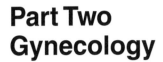

# Part Two
# Gynecology

# 39 Keys to Survival

*Keys to survival on gynecology rotations*

## WARDS

- **Common inpatient gynecology problems** (see individual chapters)
  - Postoperative care
  - PID
  - Ectopic pregnancy
- **Common floor calls**
  - *Diet*
    - Clear liquids when positive bowel sounds, solids with flatus
    - More rapid feeding is often well tolerated
  - *Analgesics* (commonly prescribed medications):
    - Oral narcotic combinations
      - Oxycodone (Percocet, 5 mg/acetaminophen, 325 mg), 1–2 PO q4–6h
      - Tylenol #3 (acetaminophen, 300 mg/codeine, 30 mg), 1–2 PO q4–6h
      - Propoxyphene (Darvocet N50, 50 mg/acetaminophen, 325 mg), 2 PO q4h
    - Nonnarcotic analgesics
      - Ibuprofen, 400–800 mg PO q6h
      - Acetaminophen (Tylenol), 650 mg PO/PR q4h
      - Ketorolac (Toradol), 30 mg IV/IM q6h or 10 mg PO q4–6h
    - IV narcotics
      - Morphine sulfate, 2–4 mg IV q2–4h
      - Hydromorphone (Dilaudid), 1–2 mg IM/SC/IV q4–6h
  - IV fluids
    - D5 half normal saline at 125 cc/hr
    - Patients who are NPO should have fluid containing dextrose

- *Decreased urine output*
  - Dehydration (increased specific gravity): bolus IV fluid (1 L normal saline over 2 hrs)
  - Blood loss (check CBC)
  - Foley catheter clotted (flush catheter or replace)
- *Ambulation*
  - Continue DVT/pulmonary embolism prophylaxis until ambulating and ready for discharge
  - Fever (see Postoperative Complications)
  - Nausea and vomiting (see Postoperative Complications)

## PREOP EVALUATION
### Review Labs

- Electrolytes (especially potassium)
  - Type and screen (make sure current)
  - Preop antibiotics (see Chap. 40, Preoperative Evaluation)
- Thromboguards or prophylactic heparin (5000 units SC bid)

## OPERATING ROOM

- Review procedure before OR
- Review anatomy
- Know common complications

## STANDARD POSTOP ORDERS
See Table 39-1.

## EMERGENCY ROOM

- **Common consults** (see individual chapters):
  - Vaginal bleeding
  - Pelvic pain
  - Rule out ectopic pregnancy
- *History*
  - Past gynecologic history: last menstrual period, STDs, contraception, number of partners
  - Past obstetric history
- *Physical exam*
  - Speculum exam

## TABLE 39-1.
## STANDARD POSTOP ORDERS

Admit: floor/attending name

Diagnosis: s/p, name of procedure, comorbidities

Condition: stable

Diet: NPO (may eat if laparoscopy)

All:

Activity: bed rest (may ambulate if minor/laparoscopy)

Vitals: q1 × 4 hrs, then q4h

Accurate input/output

IVF: D5 half normal saline tra 125 cc/hr

Foley catheter to gravity

Thromboguards to bilateral lower extremities

Incentive spirometer to bedside; teach and encourage use

Patient-controlled analgesia: standardized order sheet or

- $MSO_4$, 1 mg dose
- Lockout time: 10 mins
- Max, six doses in 1 hr
- Labs: CBC in a.m.

Meds:

- Diphenhydramine (Benadryl), 25 mg IV qhs prn
- Antiemetic (e.g., prochlorperazine [Compazine], 10 mg IV q6h prn)
- Milk of magnesia prn

Call house officer: temperature >38.2, SBP >160, or <90; DBP >110 or <40; pulse >110, respiratory rate >32, urinary output <240 cc/8 hrs

---

- Bimanual exam
  - Cervical motion tenderness
  - Adnexal tenderness masses
- Review transvaginal U/S
- Review algorithm for diagnosis/treatment of ectopic pregnancy
- **Ruptured ectopic pregnancy is a surgical emergency**
  - Call for OR
  - 2 IV lines
  - Type and cross for transfusion
- **Do not be afraid to ask your senior resident for help**

# 40

# Preoperative Evaluation

*A thorough preoperative evaluation prevents postoperative complications*

## INFORMED CONSENT

- Infectious complications of blood transfusions:
  - Fatal hemolytic reaction (1 in 100,000)
  - Nonfatal hemolytic reaction (1 in 6000)
  - HIV (1 in 493,000)
  - Hepatitis C (1 in 103,000)
  - Hepatitis B (1 in 63,000)

## CARDIOVASCULAR
### Bacterial Endocarditis Prophylaxis

- Prevents bacteremia that may seed cardiac valves
- American College of Cardiology divides patients into three risk categories (Table 40-1) [1].
- High- and moderate-risk patients warrant prophylaxis when undergoing procedures listed in Table 40-2.
- Patients undergoing c-section do not require antibiotics.
- Antibiotics are not required for vaginal hysterectomy or normal vaginal delivery but may be considered in high-risk patients.
- Antibiotic regimens listed in Table 40-3.

### Periop Beta Blockers

- Consider in patients with CAD or multiple cardiovascular risk factors
- Therapy started 1–2 wks before surgery and continued 2 wks postop
- Goal: heart rate <70 (preop), heart rate <80 (postop) [2]

## ANTICOAGULATION

- Discontinue coumadin and begin IV heparin several days before surgery.
- Heparin discontinued 48 hrs preop and resumed postop when safe.
- Coumadin then reinstituted.

**TABLE 40-1.**
**RISK STRATIFICATION FOR BACTERIAL ENDOCARDITIS**

High-risk category

    Prosthetic heart valves

    Previous endocarditis

    Complex cyanotic congenital heart disease

    Surgically constructed systemic-pulmonary shunt

Moderate-risk category

    Most other congenital cardiac malformations

    Acquired valvular heart disease

    Hypertrophic cardiomyopathy

    Mitral valve prolapse with mitral regurgitation or thickened leaflet

Low-risk category

    Isolated secundum atrial septal defect

    Surgical repair of atrial septal defect, ventricular septal defect, or patent ductus arteriosus

    Previous coronary artery bypass graft

    Mitral valve prolapse without mitral regurgitation

    Physiologic/functional murmur

    Previous Kawasaki disease without valvular disease

    Cardiac pacemaker or defibrillator

Adapted from ACC/AHA Guidelines for the management of patients with valvular heart disease. A report of the American College of Cardiology/American Heart Association. Task Force on Practice Guidelines (Committee on Management of Patients with Valvular Heart Disease). *J Am Coll Cardiol* 1998;32: 1486–1588.

- Alternative: discontinue coumadin 1–3 d preop and resume several days postop

## ANTIBIOTIC PROPHYLAXIS

Table 40.4 outlines ACOG recommendations for prophylaxis [3].

## VENOUS THROMBOEMBOLISM

- Pulmonary emboli occur in 0.1–5% of patients.

- Mortality, 10–20%.

- Most events occur within 7 d postop; increased risk remains for 3 wks.

**TABLE 40-2.**
**RECOMMENDATIONS FOR BACTERIAL**
**ENDOCARDITIS PROPHYLAXIS**

A. Endocarditis prophylaxis recommended

    Respiratory tract procedures

    GI tract procedures (optional for moderate risk)

    Genitourinary tract procedures

        Cystoscopy

        Urethral dilation

B. Endocarditis prophylaxis not recommended

    Minor respiratory procedures

        Intubation

        Bronchoscopy

    Minor GI procedures

        Endoscopy

        TEE

    Genitourinary tract procedures

        Vaginal hysterectomy (prophylaxis optional for high-risk patients)

        Vaginal delivery (prophylaxis optional for high-risk patients)

        C-section

    In uninfected tissue:

        Urethral catheterization

        Dilation and curettage

        Therapeutic abortion

        Sterilization

        Insertion/removal of IUD

    Other

    Incisional biopsy

    Circumcision

Adapted from ACC/AHA Guidelines for the management of patients with valvular heart disease. A report of the American College of Cardiology/American Heart Association. Task Force on Practice Guidelines (Committee on Management of Patients with Valvular Heart Disease). *J Am Coll Cardiol* 1998;32: 1486–1588.

**TABLE 40-3.**
**ACC/AHA REGIMENS FOR BACTERIAL**
**ENDOCARDITIS PROPHYLAXIS**

| | |
|---|---|
| High-risk patients | Ampicillin, 2 g IM/IV within 30 mins of start |
| | Gentamicin, 1.5 mg/kg IV/IM within 30 mins of start |
| | Ampicillin, 1 g IM/IV 6 hrs later |
| High risk (ampi-cillin allergy) | Vancomycin, 1 g IV complete 30 mins before start |
| | Gentamicin, 1.5 mg/kg IV/IM within 30 mins of start |
| Moderate risk | Amoxicillin, 2 g PO 1 hr before procedure or ampicillin, 3 g IV/IM within 30 mins of start |
| Moderate risk (ampicillin allergy) | Vancomycin, 1 g IV complete 30 mins before start |

Adapted from ACC/AHA Guidelines for the management of patients with valvular heart disease. A report of the American College of Cardiology/American Heart Association. Task Force on Practice Guidelines (Committee on Management of Patients with Valvular Heart Disease). *J Am Coll Cardiol* 1998;32: 1486–1588.

**TABLE 40-4.**
**ACOG RECOMMENDATIONS FOR**
**ANTIMICROBIAL PROPHYLAXIS**

| | |
|---|---|
| Vaginal/abdominal hysterec-tomy (administered just before induction of anesthesia) | Cefazolin, 1–2 g IV single dose |
| | Cefoxitin, 2 g IV single dose |
| | Cefotetan, 1–2 g IV single dose |
| | Metronidazole, 500 mg IV single dose |
| Hysterosalpingogram | Doxycycline, 100 mg bid PO × 5 d |
| Induced abortion/dilation and curettage | Doxycycline, 100 mg 1 hr before proce-dure and 200 mg after procedure |
| | Metronidazole, 500 mg bid PO for 5 d |
| Laparoscopy/hysteroscopy/lap-arotomy | None |
| Urodynamics | None |
| Endometrial biopsy/IUD | None |

Adapted from the American College of Obstetricians and Gynecologists. *Antibiotic prophylaxis for gynecologic procedures. ACOG Practice Bulletin 23.* Washington, DC: ACOG Practice Bulletin 23, 2001.

- Risk factors: malignant disease, prior venous thromboembolism, anesthesia for >5 hrs, prior abdominopelvic radiation, venous stasis, obesity, older age, and history of hereditary thrombophilia

- Prophylaxis: place before induction of anesthesia and continue 7 d or until discharge

- Thigh-high graduated compression stockings reduce DVT in medium-risk patients

- **Pneumatic compression devices:** reduce DVT in medium- and high-risk patients

- **Low-dose unfractionated heparin:** 5000 units bid or tid with dose administered 2 hrs preop

- **LMWH:** enoxaparin (Lovenox), 40 mg qd or dalteparin (Fragmin), 2500–5000 units daily

## BOWEL PREPARATION

- Administered if GI tract may be entered (Table 40-5)

- Oral GI tract lavage solutions: ingested day before surgery:

  - GoLYTELY, 1 L/hr for a maximum of 4 L until diarrheal effluent

  - Magnesium citrate, 1–2 bottles

## TABLE 40-5.
## WASHINGTON UNIVERSITY DIVISION OF GYNECOLOGIC ONCOLOGY BOWEL PREPARATION REGIMENS

| | |
|---|---|
| 1. Day before surgery | Clear liquids, NPO after midnight |
| | Magnesium citrate, 1 bottle |
| | Antibiotic bowel prep (if bowel resection anticipated) |
| | Neomycin (Mycifradin), 1 g PO q6h × 3 doses |
| | Metronidazole, 500 mg PO q6h × 3 doses |
| Day of surgery | Saline enemas until clear |
| 2. Day before surgery | Clear liquids, NPO after midnight |
| | Phosphosoda, 1.5 oz at 11:00 and 16:00 |
| | Fleet's enema at 20:00 |
| | Antibiotic bowel prep (if bowel resection anticipated) |
| | Erythromycin (E-Mycin, E.E.S., Ery-Tab, Eryc, EryPed, Ilosone), 1 g PO q4h × 3 doses |
| | Neomycin, 1 g PO q4h × 3 doses |
| Day of surgery | Soap suds enemas until clear |

- Antibiotic preparations: may be used to reduce GI tract flora
- Enemas: may be given the evening before or on day of surgery

## CORTICOSTEROIDS

- Patients treated with chronic steroids require stress dose steroids periop.
- Hydrocortisone (Cortef, Hydrocortone), 100 mg on the evening of surgery then q8h × 24 hrs.

## DIABETES MELLITUS
### Insulin Dependent

- Administer one-third to one-half neutral protamine Hagedorn insulin dose on day of surgery.
- Intraop IV dextrose with insulin supplementation.
- Sliding scale insulin postop until tolerating regular diet.

### Non–Insulin Dependent

- Stop oral hypoglycemics the day before surgery.
- Sliding scale insulin used postop until tolerating regular diet.

## REFERENCES

1. ACC/AHA Guidelines for the management of patients with valvular heart disease. A report of the American College of Cardiology/American Heart Association. Task Force on Practice Guidelines (Committee on Management of Patients with Valvular Heart Disease). *J Am Coll Cardiol* 1998;32:1486–1588.
2. Mangano DT, et al. Effect of atenolol on mortality and cardiovascular morbidity after noncardiac surgery. *N Engl J Med* 1996;335:1713–1720.
3. American College of Obstetricians and Gynecologists. *Antibiotic prophylaxis for gynecologic procedures. ACOG Practice Bulletin 23.* Washington, DC: ACOG, 2001.

# 41 Principles of Gynecologic Surgery

*General principles of gynecologic surgery*

## SUTURES
See Table 41-1.

## SKIN INCISIONS
### Pfannenstiel Incision

- Low transverse abdominal incision
- Rectus muscles separated in the midline and peritoneum opened vertically
- Good wound security, cosmesis
- Exposure limited
- Skin staples removed postop day 4–7

### Midline Incision

- Excellent exposure, rapid entry
- Hernias and dehiscences are more common
- Skin staples removed postoperative day 7–10

### Maylard Incision

- Transverse incision, rectus muscles incised transversely.
- Good pelvic exposure.

### Cherney Incision

- Transverse skin incision, rectus muscles transected at symphysis
- Good exposure to the space of Retzius

## WOUND HEALING

- **First intention:** tissue reapproximated
- **Second intention:** the wound left open to granulate
  - Used in contaminated or infected cases
- **Third intention:** (delayed primary closure)
  - Wound closed after period of being left open

## TABLE 41-1.
## COMMONLY USED SUTURES

| | |
|---|---|
| Natural absorbable sutures | Moderate tissue reaction |
|   Plain catgut | Composed of purified collagen |
| | 70% tensile strength lost in 7 d |
| | Uses: postpartum tubal ligation |
|   Chromic catgut | Catgut treated with chromic salts |
| | 50% tensile strength lost in 7–10 d |
| | Uses: hysterectomies, c-section, episiotomy |
| Synthetic absorbable sutures | Less tissue reaction, used if infection |
|   Polyglactin 910 (Vicryl) and polyglycolic acid (Dexon) | Braided filaments of synthetic fibers |
| | 50–60% of tensile strength retained at 14 d |
|   Polydioxanone (PDS) and polyglyconate (Maxon) | Monofilaments |
| | 80% tensile strength maintained at 2 wks |
| Nonabsorbable suture | Silk, polyester, polypropylene, metal |
| | Uses: cerclage (Mersilene) |

## WOUND CLOSURE

- **Fascia:** never regains original strength
  - Delayed absorbable or nonabsorbable suture used for closure
- **Mass closure:** single-layer closure through fascia, rectus muscle, and peritoneum
- **Smead-Jones retention sutures:** single-layer closure with one pass through both layers of fascia, rectus muscle, and peritoneum and a second pass through only the anterior fascia

## NERVE INJURIES

- Improper positioning can cause neurologic injury to the patient.
- **Sciatic nerve injury:** excess abduction and hyperflexion of the thigh against the abdomen in exaggerated dorsal lithotomy position.
  - Foot drop with motor and sensory loss in posterior lateral lower leg and foot
- **Peroneal nerve injury:** external rotation of leg against operative stirrups with pressure on fibular head.
  - Inability to abduct or evert the foot

- **Femoral nerve injury:** excessive lateral traction of self-retaining retractors on psoas muscle and femoral nerve.

  - Numbness over anterior thigh and difficult leg flexion and knee extension

- **Obturator nerve injury:** occurs in radical pelvic surgery, deep pelvic lymph node dissections, and retropubic urethropexy.

  - Sensory loss over medial aspect of thigh with difficult adduction

## SUGGESTED READING

Lipscomb GH, Ling FW. Wound healing, suture material and surgical instrumentation. In: Rock JA, Thompson JD, ed. *TeLinde's operative gynecology*, 8th ed. Philadelphia: Lippincott–Raven, 1997: 263–317.

# 42
# Abnormal Uterine Bleeding

*Abnormal uterine bleeding is a common gynecologic problem*

## INTRODUCTION

- Abnormal uterine bleeding characterized:
  - **Menorrhagia:** prolonged (>7 d) or heavy (>80 mL) menses
  - **Metrorrhagia:** irregular bleeding
  - **Menometrorrhagia:** prolonged or heavy menses with irregular bleeding
  - **Polymenorrhea:** menses at intervals less than 21 d

## DIFFERENTIAL DIAGNOSIS

Divided into organic lesions and dysfunctional uterine bleeding (Tables 42-1 and 42-2)

### Dysfunctional Uterine Bleeding

- Most common cause of abnormal uterine bleeding in adolescents, perimenopausal
- Endocrine cause of bleeding
- 90% of patients with dysfunctional uterine bleeding are anovulatory
- Pathology: continuous estrogenic stimulation of endometrium with irregular sloughing
- Diagnosis of exclusion

## HISTORY

- Menstrual history (amount, duration, pain)
- Menstrual calendar (pad counts)
- Basal body temperature chart (evaluate ovulation)
- Trauma

## PHYSICAL EXAM

- Pelvic exam
- Rectal exam (rule out GI bleeding)
- Speculum exam

## TABLE 42-1.
## DIFFERENTIAL DIAGNOSIS OF ABNORMAL
## UTERINE BLEEDING

**Organic causes**

1. *Genital tract pathology*

    Pregnancy complications

        Abortion (complete, incomplete, threatened)

        Ectopic pregnancy

        Molar pregnancy

    Malignancy

        Cervical cancer

        Endometrial cancer and hyperplasia

        Ovarian cancer

        Vulvar/vaginal cancer

    Infection

        PID

        Cervicitis

        Vulvovaginitis

    Trauma

    Foreign body

    Polyps (cervical, endometrial)

    Leiomyomas

    Adenomyosis

2. *Systemic diseases*

    Coagulopathies

    Blood dyscrasias

    Drugs

    Liver disease (cirrhosis)

    Hypothyroidism

**Dysfunctional uterine bleeding**

*Anovulatory*

    Eating disorders

    Excessive excercise

    PCOS

    Obesity

    Androgen excess

*Ovulatory*

## TABLE 42-2.
## DIFFERENTIAL DIAGNOSIS OF ABNORMAL UTERINE BLEEDING BY AGE GROUP

| Prepubertal | Adolescent | Reproduc-tive | Perimeno-pausal | Postmeno-pausal |
| --- | --- | --- | --- | --- |
| Vulvo-vaginitis | Anovulation | Pregnancy | Anovulation | Endometrial lesions |
| Foreign body | Pregnancy | Anovulation | Leiomyomas | Exogenous hor-mones |
| Precocious puberty | Exogenous hormones | Leiomyomas | Polyps | Atrophic vaginitis |
| Neoplasms | Coagulopa-thy | Polyps | Thyroid dis-ease | Other neoplasms |
| | | Thyroid dis-ease | | |

Reprinted from Berek JS, Adashi EY, Hillard PA, eds. *Novak's gynecology*, 12th ed. Philadelphia: Williams & Wilkins, 1996:333, with permission.

### DIAGNOSTIC EVALUATION

- Tailored by patient's age and complaints
- Pap smear
- Cervical cultures (*Gonorrhea, Chlamydia*)
- Endometrial sampling
- Endocervical curettage
- Vaginal U/S possibly with saline infusion (polyps, myomas)
- Hysteroscopy (polyps, endometrial hyperplasia, myomas)
- Lab: CBC, hCG, TSH, ferritin (assess iron stores), PT, PTT, bleeding time

### MANAGEMENT

Management of acute vaginal bleeding is outlined in Table 42-3.

### Medical Management
#### Estrogens

- Used to stop acute bleeding.
- Estrogen may be administered IV in emergency setting.
- After estrogen, give a progestational agent to stabilize endometrium and allow withdrawal bleeding.
  - Conjugated estrogen, 2.5–5 mg PO q6h, or 25–40 mg IV q6h, then add medroxyprogesterone acetate (Amen, Curretab, Cycrin, Depo-Provera, Provera), 10 mg qd × 7 d

#### Progestins

- Long-term treatment of choice for dysfunctional uterine bleeding

### TABLE 42-3.
### TREATMENT OF ACUTE VAGINAL BLEEDING

Hospitalize

Lab (CBC, PT, PTT, hCG)

IV access

IV fluid hydration

Pelvic/speculum exam

Transfusion (if symptomatic)

Estrogen

    Conjugated estrogen, 25–40 mg IV q6h

    35-µg oral contraceptive pills, 2–3 pills PO bid–tid

Dilation and curettage (unremitting bleeding)

---

- Medroxyprogesterone acetate, 10 mg PO qd × 10 d each month
- Depot medroxyprogesterone acetate, 150 mg IM q1–3 mos
- Progesterone IUD every year
- Combination oral contraceptive pills

### *NSAIDs*
- Decrease menstrual cramping and bleeding.
  - Ibuprofen, 600–800 mg PO q6–8h
  - Naproxen (Aleve), 250–500 mg PO q12h
- Other agents: danazol (Danocrine), GnRH agonists, and antifibrinolytic agents

### Surgical Management
- Dilation and curettage: provides immediate relief but long-term therapy is also required
- Endometrial ablation by resection, rollerball, thermal, cryoablation
  - Used in patients with dysfunctional uterine bleeding without genital tract pathology.
  - Improvement noted in >90% of patients
- Hysterectomy: definitive therapy

### SUGGESTED READING
American College of Obstetricians and Gynecologists. *Management of anovulatory bleeding. ACOG Practice Bulletin 14*. Washington, DC: ACOG, 2000.

Stenchever MA, Droegemueller W, Herbst AL, Mishell DR. *Comprehensive gynecology*. St. Louis: Mosby, 2001.

# 43 Acute Pelvic Pain

*A surgical emergency must quickly be ruled out in women with acute pelvic pain*

## DIFFERENTIAL DIAGNOSIS

See Table 43-1. Common causes of acute pelvic pain are discussed in other topics.

### Ovarian Torsion

- Adnexal structures twist on themselves [1].

- Most common in reproductive-aged women.

- Adnexal mass predisposes patients to torsion (most commonly teratoma).

- Unilateral lower abdominal and pelvic pain, pain often comes and goes, nausea and vomiting

- Diagnosis: requires laparoscopy or laparotomy

- Transvaginal U/S + Doppler flow may evaluate ovarian blood flow

- Treatment: surgical (untwist or adnexectomy)

### Ovarian Cysts

#### Follicular Cysts

- From gonadotropin stimulation and follicle growth

- Pain from rupture

- Diagnosis: bimanual exam, vaginal U/S

- Treatment: observation or oral contraceptive pills

#### Corpus Luteum Cysts

- Normal corpus luteum undergoes a small amount of bleeding

- Hemorrhagic corpus luteal cyst may result from cyst rupture with intraperitoneal bleeding

- Pelvic pain, menstrual irregularities

- Diagnosis: bimanual exam, vaginal U/S

- Treatment: laparoscopy or laparotomy with cystectomy

**TABLE 43-1.**
**DIFFERENTIAL DIAGNOSIS OF ACUTE PELVIC PAIN**

| | |
|---|---|
| Pregnancy related | GI |
|   Abortion |   Appendicitis |
|   Ectopic pregnancy |   Diverticulitis |
| Disorders of the uterus and cervix |   Cholecystitis |
|   Cervicitis |   Cholelithiasis |
|   Endometritis |   Gastroenteritis |
|   Degenerating myoma |   Bowel obstruction |
| Disorders of the adnexa |   Inflammatory bowel disease |
|   Salpingitis |   Irritable bowel syndrome |
|   Tuboovarian abscess |   Pancreatitis |
|   Endometriosis/endometrioma | Miscellaneous |
|   Torsion | Musculoskeletal disorders |
|   Ruptured follicular/corpus luteal cyst | Hernia |
|   Ovarian hyperstimulation | Acute porphyria |
|   Degenerating ovarian tumor | |
| Genitourinary | |
|   Cystitis | |
|   Pyelonephritis | |
|   Nephrolithiasis | |

Reprinted from Stenchever MA, Droegemueller W, Herbst AL, Mishell DR. *Comprehensive gynecology*, 4th ed. St. Louis: Mosby, 2001:162.

### Theca Lutein Cysts

- Occur during pregnancy from gonadotropin stimulation
- Often bilateral
- Treatment: observation

### HISTORY

- Pain (onset, quality, duration, location, exacerbating/relieving factors)
- Last menstrual period (normal, q28d with 3–5 d of bleeding)
- Fever or chills (temperature >38.3°C or 100.9°F)
- Nausea and vomiting, appetite, bowel movements, hematochezia, melena

- Urinary symptoms (dysuria, frequency, urgency, hematuria)
- Vaginal bleeding

## PHYSICAL EXAM

- Abdominal exam (guarding, rebound, area of tenderness)
- Pelvic exam (adnexal or cervical motion tenderness, masses)
- Speculum exam (bleeding)

## LAB EVALUATION

- CBC
- Electrolytes
- PT, PTT
- UA
- hCG
- Amylase, lipase, LFTs

## IMAGING

- Vaginal U/S
- CT of abdomen and pelvis
- Obstructive series
- IV pyelogram

## SUGGESTED READING

Stenchever MA, Droegemueller W, Herbst AL, Mishell DR. *Comprehensive gynecology.* St. Louis: Mosby, 2001.

## REFERENCE

1. Argenta PA, Yeagley TJ, Ott G, et al. Torsion of the uterine adnexa: pathologic correlations and current management trends. *J Repro Med* 2000;45:831–836.

# 44 Dysmenorrhea

*Dysmenorrhea can be debilitating*

## INTRODUCTION

- Cyclic lower abdominal cramping during or just before menses
- Classified as primary or secondary

## PRIMARY DYSMENORRHEA

- Dysmenorrhea in the absence of pelvic pathology
- Onset near menarche

### Etiology

Associated with elevated prostaglandin $F_2$-alpha levels

### History

- Cramping abdominal pain before or at onset of menses.
- Back pain, nausea, headaches, diarrhea may occur.

### Physical Exam

- Often normal
- Pelvic exam: uterine tenderness at time of dysmenorrhea

### Management

- NSAIDs
- First-line treatment
- Scheduled doses:
  - Ibuprofen (Motrin), 600–800 mg PO q6–8h
  - Naproxen (Naprosyn, Aleve), 250–500 mg bid
  - Oral contraceptive pills (may administer continuously)
- Follow-up: 3 mos

## SECONDARY DYSMENORRHEA

- Dysmenorrhea caused by underlying pelvic disease or condition
- Onset anytime in life

## TABLE 44-1.
## DIFFERENTIAL DIAGNOSIS OF
## SECONDARY DYSMENORRHEA

Cervical stenosis

Endometriosis

Transverse vaginal septum

Ovarian remnant syndrome

Imperforate hymen

Adenomyosis

Pelvic infections

Adhesions

Leiomyomas

- Table 44-1 lists conditions associated with secondary dysmenorrhea.

- Management based on underlying diagnosis.

### SUGGESTED READING

Stenchever MA, Droegemueller W, Herbst AL, Mishell DR. *Comprehensive gynecology.* St. Louis: Mosby, 2001.

# 45 Chronic Pelvic Pain

*Chronic pelvic pain is frustrating for patients and clinicians*

## INTRODUCTION

Pelvic pain for >6 mos [1]

## DIFFERENTIAL DIAGNOSIS

- Includes gynecologic and nongynecologic entities (Table 45-1).
- Psychological factors play an important role in perception of chronic pelvic pain.

### Gynecologic Causes

- Pelvic congestion: results from dilation of pelvic veins
  - Treatment: hysterectomy or embolization
- Adhesions: result from previous surgery or infection
  - Treatment: adhesiolysis
- Ovarian remnant syndrome: fragment of ovarian tissue left in place after oophorectomy
  - Diagnosis: suppressed FSH (low serum FSH)
  - Treatment: surgical excision
- Adenomyosis: endometrial tissue in myometrium
  - Treatment: hysterectomy

### GI Causes

- Irritable bowel syndrome (IBS): functional disorder with altered bowel habits
  - Treatment: depends on prominent symptoms
- Diverticulosis: outpouchings from the colonic wall
  - Acute inflammation results in diverticulitis

### Urologic Causes

- Interstitial cystitis: urgency, bladder discomfort, pain associated with bladder filling
  - Diagnosis: cystoscopy or based on symptoms

**TABLE 45-1.**
**DIFFERENTIAL DIAGNOSIS OF CHRONIC PELVIC PAIN**

| Gynecologic | GI |
|---|---|
| Endometriosis | Cholelithiasis |
| Pelvic infections | Irritable bowel syndrome |
| Leiomyoma | Inflammatory bowel disease |
| Adhesions | Diverticulosis |
| Adenomyosis | Peptic ulcer disease |
| Pelvic congestion | Chronic appendicitis |
| Ovarian remnant | Colorectal carcinoma |
| Musculoskeletal | Psychological |
| Nerve entrapment | Depression |
| Myofascial pain | Somatization |
| Arthritis | Physical abuse |
| Disk disease | Sexual abuse |
| Hernia | Substance abuse |
| Scoliosis | |
| Urologic | |
| Interstitial cystitis | |
| Urethral syndrome | |
| UTI | |
| Nephrolithiasis | |
| Detrusor overactivity | |

- Treatment: pentosan polysulfate sodium (Elmiron), 100 mg PO tid, or intravesical dimethyl sulfoxide
- Urethral syndrome: dysuria, frequency, urgency after intercourse with negative urine culture

**Musculoskeletal Causes**

- Myofascial pain: pain or spasm in areas overlying muscles may induce
  - Common muscles: obturator internus, levators, piriformis
  - Treatment: physical therapy
- Nerve entrapment: entrapment of genitofemoral or ilioinguinal nerve often after Pfannenstiel incision

- Treatment: local 1% lidocaine injections

## HISTORY

- Pain (location, quality, onset, radiation, modifiers)
- Menstrual history
- Bowel habits
- Urinary symptoms
- Surgeries
- Infections
- Physical/sexual abuse
- Depression/fatigue
- Social history

## PHYSICAL EXAM

- Abdomen (pain, scars, hernias, bowel sounds)
- Vaginal exam (masses, pain)
- Rectovaginal exam (guaiac, uterosacral nodularity)
- Trigger points (obturator internus, levator ani)
- Musculoskeletal and neurologic exams

## DIAGNOSTIC EVALUATION

- Guided by history
- Gonorrhea/chlamydia cultures
- Psychological testing (Minnesota Multiphasic Personality Inventory, Beck inventory)
- Lab: CBC, UA, urine culture, ESR, C-reactive protein (inflammation)
- Imaging: U/S, CT
- Laparoscopy

## MANAGEMENT

- Guided by likely history
- If no obvious etiology is discovered, consider laparoscopy
- 40% of patients who undergo laparoscopy have no evidence of pathology
- If endometriosis suspected, consider empiric GnRH agonist treatment if no response to oral contraceptive pills

- Psychological counseling valuable adjunct [2]

- Referral: inflammatory bowel disease, colorectal cancer, psychiatric disorders

## REFERENCES

1. Scialli AR, Barbieri RL, Olive DL, et al. Association of professors of gynecology and obstetrics educational series. *Chronic pelvic pain: an integrated approach.* Washington, DC: APGO, 2000.
2. Ling FW, for the Pelvic Pain Study Group. Randomized controlled trial of depot leuprolide in patients with chronic pelvic pain and clinically suspected endometriosis. *Obstet Gynecol* 1999;93:51–58.

# 46

# Leiomyoma

*Fibroids are very common*

## INTRODUCTION

- Also called fibroids and myomas
- Benign smooth muscle tumor
- Incidence: 25% of reproductive age women
- Risk factors: reproductive age, estrogen (obesity), black race
- Estrogen stimulates growth

## PATHOLOGY

- Histology: sharply demarcated, whorled bundles of smooth muscle
- Location: uterine corpus most common, may occur in uterine ligaments, lower uterine segment, or cervix
  - May be subserosal, submucosal, or intramural
- Degenerative changes
  - Red (carneous) degeneration occurs secondary to infarction and results in acute pain
  - Malignant (sarcomatous) degeneration in <1% [1]
- Benign variants
  - **IV leiomyomatosis:** benign smooth muscle invades vascular channels
  - **Leiomyomatosis peritonealis:** dissemination of benign nodules into peritoneal cavity
  - **Benign metastasizing leiomyoma:** benign uterine leiomyomas spread to distant sites

## HISTORY

- Abnormal uterine bleeding
- Pelvic pain, pressure
- Dysmenorrhea
- Constipation

- Urinary frequency
- Infertility
- Spontaneous abortion

## PHYSICAL EXAM

- Abdominal and pelvic examination (assess size, location, number of adnexal masses)
- Rectal exam

## DIAGNOSTIC EVALUATION

- Usually made by pelvic exam
- Optional imaging studies: pelvic U/S, CT, MRI, hysteroscopy
- Endometrial sampling in patients bleeding
- Lab: CBC, complete metabolic panel

## MANAGEMENT
### Surgical

- Hysterectomy: definitive treatment
- Myomectomy: for patients who desire future childbearing
  - Hysteroscopy, laprascopy, laparotomy

### Medical

- GnRH agonists: suppress FSH, LH resulting in hypogonadotropic hypogonadal state [2]
  - Myomas decrease in size (often 50% after 3 mos of treatment)
  - Myomas return to original size by 3 mos after cessation of treatment
  - Consider preop for large myomas or heavy bleeding
  - Leuprolide (Lupron), 3.75 mg IM every month
- Depot: depomedroxyprogesterone acetate (Depo-Provera)
- Androgens: decrease size (regrowth common)
  - Androgenic side effects

## ALTERNATIVE MANAGEMENT

- Uterine artery embolization
  - 40–70% reduction in size of myomas
  - Success rates 85–98%
  - Pain from necrosis common after procedure [3,4]

## REFERENCES

1. Leibsohn S, d'Ablaing G, Mishell DR Jr, et al. Leiomyosarcoma in a series of hysterectomies performed for resumed uterine leiomyomas. *Am J Obstet Gynecol* 1990;162:968–974.
2. Chavez NF, Stewart EA. Medical treatment of uterine fibroids. *Clin Obstet Gynecol* 2001;44(2):372–384.
3. Ravina J, Herbreteau D, Ciraru-Vigneron N. Arterial embolisation to treat uterine myomata. *Lancet* 1995;346:671–672.
4. Goodwin SC, Wong GCH. Uterine artery embolization for uterine fibroids: a radiologist's perspective. *Clin Obstet Gynecol* 2001; 44(2):412–424.

# 47

# Ectopic Pregnancy

*Ectopic pregnancy can be a life-threatening emergency*

## INTRODUCTION

- Implantation of fertilized ovum outside of uterus
- Incidence: 16/1000
- Fatality rate: 3.8/10,000 ectopic pregnancies
- 95–97% occur in fallopian tube (ampulla and isthmus most common)
- Combined intrauterine and extrauterine pregnancies (heterotopic): 1 in 30,000 gestations

## RISK FACTORS

- **Tubal damage:** PID, salpingitis isthmica nodosa, prior tubal surgery, diethylstilbestrol exposure, previous ectopic pregnancy
- **Contraception failure:** failed tubal ligation, pregnant with IUD
- **Infertility:** clomiphene, human menopausal gonadotropins, *in vitro* fertilization

## HISTORY

- Abdominal pain (90–100%)
- Pain referred to shoulder (diaphragm irritation from hemoperitoneum)
- Amenorrhea (75–95%)
- Vaginal bleeding (50–80%)
- Syncope (20–35%)

## PHYSICAL EXAM

- Vital signs (tachycardia, hypotension, orthostatics, fever [5–10%])
- Abdominal tenderness (70–95%, guarding, rebound)
- Pelvic exam: adnexal mass (palpable in 50%)

## DIAGNOSTIC EVALUATION

See Fig. 47-1.

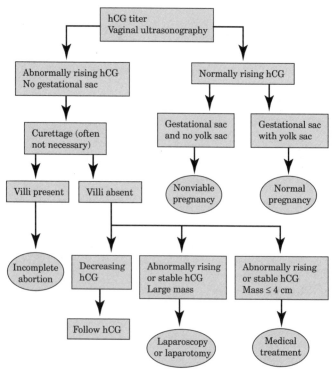

**FIG. 47-1.**
Evaluation and treatment of suspected ectopic pregnancy. (Reprinted from Speroff L, Glass RH, Kase NG. *Clinical gynecologic endocrinology and infertility*, 6th ed. Baltimore: Lippincott Williams & Wilkins 1999:1157, with permission.)

## Quantitative hCG

• Most ectopic pregnancies have lower hCG than intrauterine pregnancies (IUPs)

• Normal pregnancies have 66% increase in hCG q48h

• Abnormal pregnancies (nonviable IUP, ectopics) do not have similar increase in hCG

• Serial hCG measurements (q48h) followed to diagnosis ectopic pregnancy

## Ultrasound

• Identifying IUP by U/S rules out an ectopic gestation

- IUP visualized at hCG levels:
  - 1000–2000 mIU/mL by transvaginal U/S
  - 6500 mIU/mL by transabdominal U/S
- Earliest evidence of IUP is an intrauterine gestational sac
- Double decidual sign specific for IUP
- Sonographic findings of ectopic pregnancy: free fluid, adnexal mass, extrauterine embryo, adnexal ring

## Uterine Curettage

- Performed if plateau or decline in hCG level
- Chorionic villi confirm nonviable IUP and rule out ectopic pregnancy

## Progesterone

- Level <5 mg/mL identifies nonviable gestation with 100% specificity.

## Culdocentesis

- Aspirating fluid from the posterior cul-de-sac through posterior vaginal wall
- Nonclotting blood aids diagnosis (70–90% of ectopics have positive culdocentesis)
- Now infrequently performed because of ultrasound

## Laparoscopy

- Definitive method of diagnosis

## MANAGEMENT
### Surgical

- Linear salpingostomy (procedure of choice) or salpingectomy
- Hemodynamically stable patients candidates for laparoscopy

## Medical

- Single-dose methotrexate successful in 80–90% of patients [2,3].
- Decline of 15% in hCG should be noted between days 4 and 7 after administration.
- Protocol for methotrexate outlined in Appendix H. 6
- Contraindications listed in Table 47-1.
- All Rh (–) patients require Rh immunoglobulin (RhoGAM).

**TABLE 47-1.**
## CONTRAINDICATIONS TO METHOTREXATE

| Absolute | Relative |
|---|---|
| Hemodynamically unstable | Gestational sac > 3.5 cm |
| Breastfeeding | Embryonic cardiac activity |
| Immunodeficiency | hCG >15,000 mIU/mL |
| Liver disease | Poor compliance to follow-up |
| Alcoholism | |
| Blood dyscrasia | |
| Peptic ulcer disease | |
| Renal dysfunction | |
| Sensitivity to methotrexate | |

## PROGNOSIS

- Weekly hCG measurements to rule out **persistent ectopic pregnancy**
  - 5% after laporotomy, 15% after laparoscopy
- 85% of patients will have a normal gestation during next pregnancy
- Recurrent ectopic pregnancy occurs in 10–20% of patients

## REFERENCES

1. American College of Obstetricians and Gynecologists. *Medical management of tubal pregnancy. ACOG Practice Bulletin 3.* Washington DC: ACOG, 1998.
2. Lipscomb GH, Stovall TG, Ling FW. Nonsurgical treatment of ectopic pregnancy. *N Engl J Med* 2000;343:1325–1329.
3. Lipscomb GH, McCord ML, Stovall TG, et al. Predictors of success of methotrexate treatment in women with tubal ectopic pregnancies. *N Engl J Med* 1999;341:1974–1977.

# 48 Endometriosis

*Endometrial tissue outside of the uterus*

## INTRODUCTION

- Growth of endometrium outside the uterus
- Most common between ages 25 and 35 yrs
- Incidence: 10% of reproductive age women, 25–35% of infertile women

## ETIOLOGY

- Theories of etiology:
  - Retrograde menstruation (Sampson): retrograde menstruation with spread of endometrial tissue into the peritoneal cavity
  - Coelomic metaplasia: transformation of coelomic epithelium into endometrial tissue
  - Vascular/lymphatic: spread by vascular and lymphatic channels

## PATHOLOGY

- Endometrial implants composed of endometrial glands, stroma, hemorrhage
- Implants responsive to ovarian steroids
- Common location of implants: ovary, anterior and posterior cul-de-sacs, uterosacral ligaments, broad ligaments, rectosigmoid, appendix
- Endometriomas (chocolate cysts): ovarian cysts with hemorrhage and degradation

## HISTORY

- Pelvic pain
- Infertility
- Dyspareunia
- Dysmenorrhea
- Abnormal vaginal bleeding

## PHYSICAL EXAM

Pelvic exam: uterosacral nodularity, fixed or retroverted uterus, enlarged ovaries

## DIAGNOSTIC EVALUATION

- Laparoscopy: direct visualization
- U/S or MRI can identify endometriomas
- CA-125: neither sensitive nor specific; may monitor treatment

## MANAGEMENT

- Based on complaint (infertility or pain).
- Infertility: surgical treatment used.
  - Value of treating mild endometriosis to improve infertility is uncertain.
- Pain: managed initially with medical treatment [1].
- See Fig. 48-1.

### Surgical Treatment

- Conservative: laparoscopy with laser ablation, excision or fulguration of implants with lysis of adhesions [2].
- Presacral neurectomy or laprascopic uterosacral nerve ablation considered.
- Hysterectomy with bilateral salpingo-oophorectomy is definitive treatment.

### Medical Treatment

- All available agents are similar in efficacy.
- GnRH agonists: gonadotropin suppression results in hypoestrogenic state.
  - Treatment limited to 6 mos to prevent bone loss
  - Leuprolide (Lupron), 3.75 mg IM every month
  - Goserelin (Zoladex), 3.6 mg SC every month
  - Estrogen and progesterone "add back" considered
    - Add back therapy: conjugated equine estrogen, 0.625 mg, and medroxyprogesterone acetate (Provera), 2.5 mg qd
- Progestational agents: endometrial decidualization and implant atrophy.
  - Medroxyprogesterone acetate, 30 mg PO qd

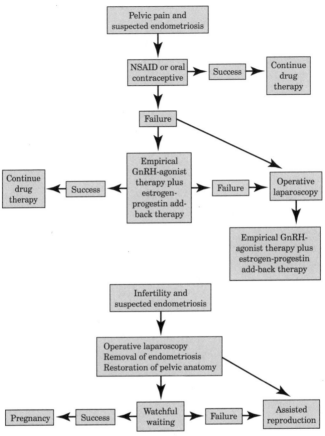

**FIG. 48-1.**
Management of endometriosis. (Reprinted from Olive DL, Pritts EA. Treatment of endometriosis. *N Engl J Med* 2001;345:266–275, with permission.)

- Oral contraceptive pills: endometrial decidualization

  - Continuous hormonal therapy without placebo interval may be beneficial.

- **Danazol:** inhibits LH and FSH surges and steroidogenesis

  - Side effects from androgenic effects

  - 400 mg PO bid

## PROGNOSIS

Recurrence common (40% at 5 yrs for medical management, 20% after surgery)

## REFERENCES

1. Olive DL, Pritts EA. Treatment of endometriosis. *N Engl J Med* 2001;345:266–275.
2. Marcoux S, Maheux R, Berube S, Canadian Collaborative Group on Endometriosis. Laprascopic surgery in infertile women with minimal or mild endometriosis. *N Engl J Med* 1997;337:217–222.

# 49

# Müllerian Anomalies

*Common müllerian anomalies*

## INTRODUCTION

- Result from abnormal fusion or canalization of müllerian ducts
- Incidence: 2–3% at time of vaginal delivery
- Classification described in Fig. 49-1

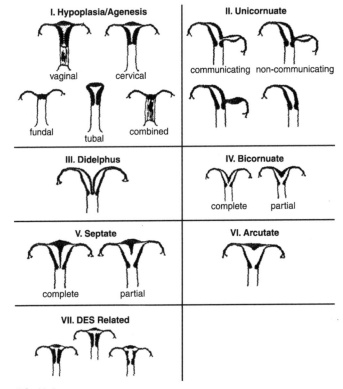

**FIG. 49-1.**
Classification of müllerian anomalies. (Reprinted from Callen PW, ed. *Ultrasonography in obstetrics and gynecology*, 4th ed. Philadelphia: WB Saunders 2000:899, with permission.)

## COMPLICATIONS

- Often asymptomatic
- Spontaneous abortion, ectopic pregnancy, preterm labor, IUGR, abnormal fetal lies, uterine rupture

## DIAGNOSIS

- Hysterosalpingogram and laparoscopy or MRI
- Women with history of DES exposure *in utero* are at increased risk of müllerian anomalies and clear cell carcinoma of the vagina [1]

## REFERENCES

1. Herbst AL, Ulfelder H, Poskanzer DC. Adenocarcinoma of the vagina: association of maternal stilbestrol therapy with tumor appearance in young women. *N Engl J Med* 1971;284:878–882.
2. Callen, PW. *Ultrasonography in obstetrics and gynecology*, 4th ed. Philadelphia: WB Saunders, 2000.

# 50 Disorders of the Vulva

*Common vulva disorders*

## BARTHOLIN'S GLAND INFECTIONS

- Bartholin's glands: openings at 5 and 7 o'clock between hymen and labia minora
- Enlargement: cyst, abscess, carcinoma

### Management

- Mildly symptomatic cysts: observation
- Abscesses/symptomatic cysts: drainage (marsupialization or Word catheter for 4–6 wks)

## NONNEOPLASTIC EPITHELIAL DISORDERS

Punch biopsies for diagnosis

### Lichen Sclerosus

- Epithelial thinning, fibrosis, and edema
- Inspection: vulva white, thin, paperlike appearance; ulcers; fissures; agglutination
- Diagnosis: biopsy
- Treatment: high-potency topical corticosteroids bid for 2–3 d, then daily until symptoms resolve (Table 50-1)

### Squamous Cell Hyperplasia

- Epithelial thickening
- Inspection: vulva gray or white lesions with acanthosis, mild hyper-keratosis
- Diagnosis: biopsy
- Treatment: medium-strength topical coritcosteroids bid until symptoms improve, then daily until symptoms resolve (Table 50-1).

## VESTIBULITIS

- Vulvodynia, dyspareunia, vulvar burning, urinary symptoms, inflammation and pressure on vestibule
- Etiology: unknown

**TABLE 50-1.**
## TOPICAL CORTICOSTEROIDS

| Corticosteroid | Strength (%) | Frequency of application |
|---|---|---|
| Very high potency | | |
|    Halobetasol propionate (Ulravate) | 0.05 | bid/tid |
|    Clobetasol propionate (Temovate) | 0.05 | qd/bid |
| High potency | | |
|    Triamcinolone (Kenalog, Aristocort) | 0.1 | tid/qid |
|    Betamethasone valerate (Valisone) | 0.1 | qd/bid |
|    Fluocinolone acetonide (Synalar) | 0.2 | qd/qid |
| Low potency | | |
|    Hydrocortisone acetate (Cortaid) | 0.5–1.0 | tid/qid |

- Treatment: TCAs, topical capsaicin, topical corticosteroids, topical anesthetics
- Resolves spontaneously in one-third of patients

### ESSENTIAL (IDIOPATHIC) VULVODYNIA

- Vulvar pain with no clear etiology
- Treatment: supportive, TCAs

### OTHER VULVAR DISEASES

- Systemic dermatoses, benign tumors, infectious diseases involving the vulva
- Biopsy vulvar lesions if uncertain

### SUGGESTED READING

Foster DC. Vulvar disease. *Obstet Gynecol* 2002;100:145–163.

Stenchever MA, Droegemueller W, Herbst AL, Mishell DR. *Comprehensive gynecology*. St. Louis: Mosby, 2001.

# 51

# Sexual Assault

*Residents should feel comfortable evaluating victims of sexual assault*

## HISTORY

- Obstetric and gynecologic history (chaperone present for support)
- STD history
- Description of assault
- Rule out acute injury

## EVIDENCE COLLECTION

- Samples of vaginal secretions, saliva, pubic hair, scalp hair, finger-nail scrapings, clothing
- Wood's lamp exam for semen
- Evidence collection kits usually available
- Preserve chain of evidence

## SCREENING AND PROPHYLAXIS

- Gonococcal infections occur in 6–12%, syphilis in 3%.
- Table 51-1 outlines recommendations.
- Rate of acquisition of HIV low; prophylaxis [1] may be offered (Table 51-2).

## PSYCHOLOGICAL EVALUATION

- May develop rape trauma syndrome
- Acute phase: individual's coping mechanisms paralyzed (hours to days)
- Organization phase: develops phobias, flashbacks (months to years)
- Social work and sexual assault counseling

## TABLE 51-1.
## INFECTIOUS DISEASE SCREENING FOR VICTIMS OF SEXUAL ASSAULT

|  | Screening | Prophylaxis |
| --- | --- | --- |
| Initial exam | Neisseria gonorrhoeae | Hepatitis B vaccine |
|  | Chlamydia trachomatis | Hepatitis immune globulin, 0.06 mL/kg IM × 1 |
|  | Wet prep (bacterial vaginosis, Candida, Trichomonas) | |
|  | hCG | Ceftriaxone (Rocephin), 125 mg IM × 1 |
| 2-wk follow up | N. gonorrhoeae | Doxycycline (Monodox, Periostat, Vibramycin), 100 mg bid × 7 d |
|  | C. trachomatis | |
|  | Wet prep (bacterial vaginosis, Candida, Trichimonas) | Metronidazole (Flagyl), 2 g PO × 1 |
|  | hCG | Emergency contraception |
|  |  | Offer HIV prophylaxis |
| 12-wk follow up | VDRL | |
|  | HIV | |
|  | Hepatitis B virus (if not vaccinated) | |

## TABLE 51-2.
## PROPHYLACTIC REGIMENS FOR HIV

Preferred regimen (28 d)

Zidovudine (Retrovir), 300 mg bid or 200 mg tid; and lamivudine (Epivir, Epivir-HBV), 150 mg bid

Alternative regimen (28 d)

Didanosine (Videx), 200 mg bid; and stavudine (Zerit), 40 mg bid

## REFERENCE

1. Bamberger JD, Waldo CR, Gerberding JL, et al. Postexposure prophylaxis for human immunodeficiency virus (HIV) infection following sexual assault. Am J Med 1999;106:323–326.

# 52 Postoperative Complications

*Postoperative complications must be recognized and treated*

## INTRODUCTION

Standard postop orders are displayed in Chap. 39, Keys to Survival

## POSTOPERATIVE FEVER

- Temp of 100.4°F (38°C) on two occasions at least 4 hrs apart, not in the first 24 hrs after surgery
- Differential diagnosis: Table 52-1

## PHYSICAL EXAM

- Vital signs, fever curve, tachycardia
- Abdominal and pelvic examinations
- Calf exam (tenderness, erythema, asymmetry)
- Wound exam (erythema, exudates, fascial integrity)

### Lab Evaluation

- Basic evaluation: CBC and UA
- Chest x-ray if pulmonary symptoms
- Optional: blood cultures, CT, lower extremity Dopplers

## DEEP VENOUS THROMBOSIS
### Physical Exam

- Erythema, pain, asymmetric calf swelling

### Diagnosis

- Duplex U/S (>90% sensitive)

### Management

- IV heparin (nomogram in appendix)
- LMWH may be substituted
- Warfarin instituted once aPTT therapeutic therapy
- Heparin continued INR 2–3 for 48 hrs

## TABLE 52-1.
## DIFFERENTIAL DIAGNOSIS OF POSTOP FEVER

| Etiology | Day of onset | Notes |
| --- | --- | --- |
| Atelectasis | 1–2 d | Most common cause of postop fever |
| | | Treatment with incentive spirometery, ambulation, prevention |
| UTI | After 3 d | Increased by prolonged indwelling catheter |
| | | Treatment: antibiotics |
| Pneumonia | After 3 d | Treatment: antibiotics |
| Superficial phlebitis | Any time | Increased if IV lines in place for > 48 hrs |
| | | Redness, pain, and induration at IV site |
| | | Treatment: change lines, warm compresses |
| Deep venous thrombosis | 3–7 d | See below |
| Wound infections | 5–10 d | Incidence <5% |
| | | Incisional pain, erythema, tenderness and drainage |
| | | Treatment: open wound, débride and dressing changes (bid wet to dry), delayed primary closure can be offered at follow-up |
| | | Rule out fascial dehiscence and necrotizing fasciitis |
| Necrotizing fasciitis | 2–10 d | Surgical emergency with 30–50% mortality |
| | | Fever, tachycardia, incisional pain, crepitus and bullae in wound |
| | | Tracks beyond superficial margin |
| | | Treatment: antibiotics, wide débridement |
| Pelvic cellulitis | 3–5 d | Soft tissue infection with inflammation at vaginal cuff |
| | | Abdominal pain, pelvic pain |
| | | Treatment: antibiotics, open vaginal cuff to allow drainage |
| Pelvic abscess | 3–5 d | Infected intraperitoneal or retroperitoneal fluid collection |
| | | Abdominal pain, pelvic pain |
| | | Treatment: antibiotics, drainage |
| Drug fever | Any time | High fever, often does not appear ill |
| | | Diagnosis of exclusion |
| | | Treatment: discontinuation of drug |

- Oral warfarin continued long term in high-risk patients, 6 mos in moderate-risk patients, and 3 mos in low-risk patients

## Complications

- Pulmonary emboli
- Postphlebitic syndrome

## PULMONARY EMBOLISM
## History

Nonspecific (dyspnea, chest pain, apprehension, cough, hemoptysis, diaphoresis)

## Physical Exam

Nonspecific (tachypnea, crackles, tachycardia, hypoxia)

## General Diagnostic Evaluation

- CBC, PT, PTT
- ABG (increased A-a gradient, hypoxemia, hypocapnia)
- ECG (tachycardia, S1Q1T3, nonspecific ST abnormalities)
- Chest x-ray (exclude other pulmonary disease, decreased vascularity, infarction)
- Echocardiogram (if hemodynamically unstable)
- Above are nonspecific, do not exclude pulmonary embolism

## Specific Diagnostic Evaluation
## $\dot{V}/\dot{Q}$ Scan

- Initial procedure of choice.
- Interpretation depends on pretest probability of pulmonary embolism.
- High-probability scan: treat for PE.
- Intermediate-probability scan/low-probability scan with a high pretest probability of pulmonary embolism: lower extremity duplex scanning or pulmonary angiogram.
  - If duplex scan positive for DVT: anticoagulation (as above).
  - If lower extremity duplex scan negative: pulmonary angiogram [1,2]

## Pulmonary Angiogram

Performed when other evaluations equivocal: considered gold standard

### Spiral (Helical) CT

- Considered in place of $\dot{V}/\dot{Q}$ scan as initial test
- Insensitive emboli below level of segmental pulmonary artery

### Management

- Supportive care: $O_2$, IV fluid
- Anticoagulation
- Begin during diagnostic evaluation
- IV heparin or LMWH initiated
- Oral warfarin instituted once aPTT therapeutic (see Appendix F)
- Thrombectomy: consider for unstable patients
- Inferior vena cava filter: patients with contraindication to anticoagulation, develop recurrent emboli while being anticoagulated

### GI COMPLICATIONS

- Postop ileus and bowel obstruction may complicate abdominal surgery.
- Patients present with N/V.
- See Table 52-2.

### TABLE 52-2.
### ILEUS AND BOWEL OBSTRUCTION

|  | Ileus | Bowel obstruction |
|---|---|---|
| Onset | 24–72 hrs postop | Delayed |
| Pain | Mild | Severe, cramping |
| Abdominal exam | Distention | Distention |
| Bowel sounds | Hypoactive | Hyperactive |
| Abdominal radiograph |  |  |
|   Bowel dilation | Small and large bowel | Proximal to obstruction |
|   Air-fluid levels | Infrequent | Usually present |
| Management | Bowel rest, nasogastric suction, antiemetics, cholinergics, enemas, fluid hydration | Medical: bowel rest, nasogastric suction, antiemetics, fluid hydration |
|  |  | Surgical |

## PAIN MANAGEMENT

- Initially: patient-controlled analgesic pump or IV narcotics
- Oral analgesics begun once tolerating oral intake

## DEHISCENCE AND EVISCERATION

- **Fascial dehiscence:** opening in the fascia
- **Evisceration:** abdominal contents protrude through the dehiscence
- Signs and symptoms: large volume serosanguinous drainage, prolonged ileus, increased patient discomfort
- Diagnosis: palpation of fascial defect
- Management: IV fluid hydration, bowel decompression with nasogastric tube, antibiotics, wound closure in OR

## SUGGESTED READING

Stenchever MA, Droegemueller W, Herbst AL, Mishell DR. *Comprehensive gynecology*. St. Louis: Mosby, 2001.

## REFERENCES

1. Goldhaber SZ. Pulmonary embolism. *N Engl J Med* 1998;339:93–104.
2. PIOPED Investigators. Value of the ventilation/perfusion scan in acute pulmonary embolism: results of the Prospective Investigation of Pulmonary Embolism Diagnosis. *JAMA* 1990;263:2753–2759.

# Gynecologic
# Infectious
# Disease

# 53 Vulvovaginitis

*Vaginal discharge is a common complaint*

## DIAGNOSTIC EVALUATION

- Speculum exam (vaginal pH, microscopy with normal saline and KOH)

- Cervical cultures (*Chlamydia trachomatis, Neisseria gonorrhoeae*)

## DIFFERENTIAL DIAGNOSIS

- Bacterial vaginosis (50%), candidiasis (25%), *Trichomonas vaginalis* (25%)

- See Table 53-1

## BACTERIAL VAGINOSIS

- Overgrowth of anaerobic bacteria and replacement vaginal lactobacilli

- *Gardnerella vaginalis* common organism found

### Diagnosis

3 of 4 criteria:

- Homogenous vaginal discharge

- pH >4.5

- Whiff test positive (amine-like odor when discharge mixed with KOH)

- Clue cells (vaginal epithelial cells with adherent bacteria) >20%

### Management

- Metronidazole (Flagyl), 500 mg PO bid × 7 d (95% cure)

- Metronidazole gel 0.75%, 1 applicator qd × 5 d

- Clindamycin (Cleocin), 2% cream, 1 applicator qhs × 7 d

## *TRICHOMONAS VAGINALIS*

- Profuse vaginal discharge with foul odor

- Vulvar pruritus and a strawberry-appearing cervix

**TABLE 53-1.**
**DIFFERENTIAL DIAGNOSIS OF VULVOVAGINITIS**

| Etiology | pH | Diagnosis | Discharge | Treatment |
|---|---|---|---|---|
| Physiologic discharge | 3.5–4.5 | — | Thin white discharge | — |
| Bacterial vaginosis | > 4.5 | Clue cells | Gray, homogenous<br><br>Whiff test (+) | Metronidazole (Flagyl), 500 mg bid × 7 d |
| Trichomonas vaginalis | 6–7 | Motile protozoa | Yellow gray, homogenous<br><br>Strawberry cervix | Metronidazole, 2 g PO × 1 |
| Candida | 4–5 | Pseudohyphae, budding hyphae | Thick, white "cottage cheese" | Topical azole<br><br>Fluconazole (Diflucan), 150 mg PO × 1 |
| Atrophic vaginitis | >4.5 | — | Inflammatory discharge | Topical estrogen |

## Diagnosis

Flagellated protozoa, WBCs on microscopy

## Management

- Metronidazole, 2 g PO × 1
- Resistant strains
  - Metronidazole, 500 mg PO bid × 7 d
  - Metronidazole, 2 g PO qd × 5 d
- Treat male partner

## *CANDIDA* VAGINITIS

- *Candida albicans* (*C. glabrata*, *C. tropicalis* less common)
- Diabetes, antibiotics, pregnancy, immunosuppression predispose
- Thick white vaginal discharge, extensive vulvar pruritus

## Diagnosis

Hyphae and spores on KOH prep

**TABLE 53-2.
ANTIFUNGAL MEDICATIONS FOR
CANDIDAL VULVOVAGINITIS**

| Medication | Dose |
|---|---|
| Oral | |
| Fluconazole (Diflucan) | 150 mg PO × 1 |
| Vaginal | |
| Butoconazole (Femstat) | 1 applicator qhs × 3 d (6 d if pregnant) |
| Clotrimazole (Mycelex, Gyne-Lotrimin) | 1 applicator qhs × 7 d |
| | 100-mg vaginal tablet qhs × 7 d |
| | 500-mg vaginal tablet × 1 |
| Miconazole (Monistat) | 1 applicator qhs × 7 d |
| | 100 mg vaginal tabs qhs × 7 d |
| | 200 mg vaginal tabs qhs × 3 d |
| Terconazole (Terazol) | 1 applicator 0.4% qhs × 7 d |
| | 1 applicator 0.8% qhs × 3 d |
| | 80 mg vaginal tab qhs × 3 d |
| Tiocazole (Vagistat, Monistat-1) | 1 applicator 6.5% cream × 1 |

## Management

- Topical azole therapy (1, 3, or 7 d) or fluconazole (Diflucan) (Table 53-2)
  - Recurrent candidal infections (> 4/yr)
  - Vaginal culture (identify *C. glabrata* or *C. tropicalis*)
  - Non-albicans species identified: fluconazole
  - Other treatments:
    - Boric acid, 600 mg intravaginally bid
    - Gentian violet painted vaginally once/wk × 4 wks
    - Ketoconazole (Nizoral), 400 mg PO qd

## ATROPHIC VAGINITIS

Thinning of vaginal epithelium due to estrogen deficiency

## Diagnosis

History and numerous WBCs on microscopy

### Management

- 0.01% estrogen, 2–4 g qd × 1–2 wks, decrease by 50% for 1–2 wks, then 1 g 1–3×/wk for maintenance therapy

- Conjugated estrogen cream, 2–4 g × 3 wks each month × 3–6 mos

### SUGGESTED READING

Centers for Disease Control. 2002 Guidelines for treatment of sexually transmitted diseases, *MMWR Morb Mortal Wkly Rep* 2002;51:1–80.

Stenchever MA, Droegemueller W, Herbst AL, Mishell DR. *Comprehensive gynecology.* St. Louis: Mosby, 2001.

# 54

# Cervicitis

*Gonorrhea and* Chlamydia *cervicitis*

## INTRODUCTION

- *Neisseria gonorrhoeae* and *Chlamydia trachomatis*
- *Chlamydia* most frequent; coinfection common

## HISTORY

- Vaginal discharge (color, quantity)
- Pruritus

## DIAGNOSTIC EVALUATION

- Mucopus in endocervix with ≥10 polymorphonuclear leukocytes/high-power field on microscopy
- Cervix friable and erythematous
- DNA probe assay or culture for *Neisseria* and *Chlamydia*
- Offer testing for syphilis, HIV, hepatitis, wet prep

## MANAGEMENT

- May presumptively treat for *N. gonorrhoeae* and *C. trachomatis* (Table 54-1).
- Azithromycin (Zithromax, Zithromax Z-Pak) with ceftriaxone most commonly used.
- Test of cure no longer recommended outside of pregnancy.

**TABLE 54-1.**
**TREATMENT OF CHLAMYDIAL AND**
**GONOCOCCAL INFECTIONS**

*Chlamydia trachomatis*

Recommended

Azithromycin (Zithromax), 1 g PO × 1

Doxycycline (Monodox, Periostat, Vibramycin), 100 mg PO bid × 7 d

Alternate

Erythromycin base (E-Mycin, EES, Ery-Tab, Eryc, EryPed, Ilosone), 500 mg PO qid × 7 d

Erythromycin ethylsuccinate (EES), 800 mg PO qid × 7 d

Ofloxacin (Floxin), 300 mg PO bid × 7 d

Levofloxacin (Levaquin), 500 mg PO qd × 7 d

*Neisseria gonorrhoeae*

Recommended

Ceftriaxone (Rocephin), 125 mg IM × 1

Cefixime (Suprax), 400 mg PO × 1

Ciprofloxacin (Cipro, Cipro XR), 500 mg PO × 1

Ofloxacin, 400 mg PO × 1

Levofloxacin, 250 mg PO × 1

Alternate

Spectinomycin (Trobicin), 2 g IM × 1

## SUGGESTED READING

Centers for Disease Control and Prevention. 2002 Guidelines for treatment of sexually transmitted diseases. *MMWR Morb Mortal Wkly Rep* 2002;51:1–80.

# 55

# Pelvic Inflammatory Disease

*PID is a major cause of infertility and ectopic pregnancy*

## INTRODUCTION

- Infection of female upper genital tract
- 1 million cases annually

## ETIOLOGY

- **Microbiology:** polymicrobial infection
- *Chlamydia trachomatis, Neisseria gonorrhoeae,* anaerobes
- Silent PID: asymptomatic infection
- **Transmission:** ascending infection from the cervix and vagina
- Uterine instrumentation increases risk

## RISK FACTORS

See Table 55-1.

## HISTORY

- Diagnosis based on clinical findings (err on side of overtreating)
- Lower abdominal pain (99%)
- Vaginal discharge (69%)
- Irregular bleeding (40%)
- Fever (34%)
- Urinary symptoms (20%)
- Vomiting (10%)

## PHYSICAL EXAM

- CDC recommends treatment if lower abdominal tenderness, adnexal tenderness, and cervical motion tenderness are present
- Vital signs [temperature >38.5°C (101.3°F)]
- Abdominal exam (lower abdominal tenderness)
- Pelvic exam (adnexal tenderness, masses, cervical motion tenderness)

**TABLE 55-1.**
**RISK FACTORS AND PROTECTIVE FACTORS FOR PID**

| Risk factors | Protective factors |
| --- | --- |
| Young age | Contraception use |
| Multiple sexual partners | Oral contraceptive pills |
| Previous PID | Barrier methods |
| No contraception use | |
| IUD (only around the time of insertion) | |
| Uterine instrumentation | |

- Speculum exam and wet prep (discharge, *C. trachomatis*, *N. gonorrhoeae*)
- Laparoscopy (gold standard for diagnosis, rarely required)

## DIAGNOSTIC EVALUATION

- Lab (hCG, UA, ESR, CRP, VDRL, HIV, HBsAg, hepatitis C)
- Leukocytosis (CBC)
- TVS (tuboovarian abscess)
- Sedimentation rate, C-reactive protein (nonspecific, rarely needed)

## DIFFERENTIAL DIAGNOSIS

- Pregnancy complications: ectopic pregnancy
- GI: appendicitis, diverticulitis, cholecystitis
- Urinary: cystitis, pyelonephritis, nephrolithiasis

## MANAGEMENT

- Determine need for hospitalization (Table 55-2)
- Antibiotics (see Table 55-2)
- Counsel: long-term sequelae, treatment of sexual partners

## COMPLICATIONS

- **Tuboovarian abscess:** adnexal abscess that results from PID.
- Often follows recurrent episodes of PID.
- Diagnosis: adnexal mass on exam, confirmed by U/S.

## TABLE 55-2.
## TREATMENT OF PID

Indications for hospitalization

    Tuboovarian abscess

    Pregnancy

    Adolescents

    Immunodeficiency (HIV)

    Uncertain diagnosis

    Surgical emergencies

    Nausea and vomiting (precluding PO treatment)

    History of operative or diagnostic procedure

    Failed outpatient treatment

    Peritonitis

    IUD

Outpatient regimen

    Doxycycline (Monodox, Periostat, Vibramycin), 100 mg PO bid × 14 d + ceftriaxone (Rocephin), 250 mg IM × 1 or cefoxitin (Mefoxin), 2 g IM × 1 + probenecid (Benemid, Probalan), 1 g PO × 1 or parenteral ceftizoxime or cefotaxime (Claforan) ± metronidazole (Flagyl), 500 mg PO bid × 14 d

Inpatient regimens

    Regimen A

        Doxycycline, 100 mg IV/PO bid + cefotetan (Cefotan), 2 g IV bid, or cefoxitin, 2 g IV q6h. Discontinue 24 hrs after clinically improved. Continue doxycycline for 14 d.

    Regimen B

        Clindamycin (Cleocin), 900 mg IV q8h

        Gentamycin (Garamycin), 2 mg/kg load, then 1.5 mg/kg q8h (or qd dosing)

- Treatment: similar to that for PID.

  - Long-term resolution may require percutaneous aspiration or operative removal.

- **Fitz-Hugh-Curtis syndrome:** perihepatic inflammation by intra-abdominal spread.

- **Long-term sequelae:** infertility, ectopic pregnancy, chronic pelvic pain [1].

## SUGGESTED READING

Centers for Disease Control and Prevention: 2002 Guidelines for treatment of sexually transmitted diseases. *MMWR Morb Mortal Wkly Rep* 2002;51:1–80.

## REFERENCE

1. Westrom L, Joesoef R, Reynolds G, et al. Pelvic inflammatory disease and fertility: a cohort study of 1,844 women with laparoscopically verified disease and 657 control women with normal laparoscopic results. *Sex Transmit Dis* 1992;19:185.

# 56

# Sexually Transmitted Diseases

*Common STDs*

## SYPHILIS

- *Treponema pallidum* (spirochete)
- Transmission: sexual contact

## Clinical Manifestations
### Primary Syphilis

- Hard, painless ulcer: chancre (vulva, vagina, cervix)
- If untreated 50% develop secondary infection; 50% develop latent syphilis

### Secondary Syphilis

- 6 wks–6 mos after chancre
- Manifestations include a maculopapular palmar/plantar rash and condyloma lata (gray white vulvar patches)

### Latent Syphilis

Positive serology without clinical manifestations

### Tertiary Syphilis

CNS (paresis, tabes dorsalis, optic atrophy), aortic aneurysms, bone gummas

## Diagnosis

- Screening: nontreponemal tests (VDRL and RPR)
- Confirmatory: treponemal tests (FTA-ABS or microhemagglutination–*T. pallidum*)

## Management
### Early Syphilis (Primary, Secondary, Latent <1 Yr)

- Benzathine penicillin G (Bicillin L-A), 2.4 million U IM × 1
- Alternate
  - Doxycycline (Monodox, Periostat, Vibramycin), 100 mg PO bid × 14 d

- Tetracycline (Achromycin, Panmycin, Sumycin, Tetracap), 500 mg PO qid × 14 d

### *Late Syphilis (Latent >1 yr, tertiary)*

- Benzathine penicillin G, 2.4 million U IM q wk × 3
- Alternate
  - Doxycycline, 100 mg PO bid × 14 d (4 wks if >1 yr)
  - Tetracycline, 500 mg PO qid × 14 d (4 wks if >1 yr)

### *Pregnant Patients*

- Treat based on stage, as above.
- Patients with penicillin allergy should be desensitized.

## HERPES SIMPLEX VIRUS
## Clinical Manifestations

- Small, painful vesicles on anogenital region.
- Vesicles ulcerate to form shallow, tender lesions.
- Initial episode most severe (often fever, myalgias, inguinal adenopathy, headache, aseptic meningitis).
- Ocular manifestations (blepharitis, keratitis, and kerotoconjunctivitis), meningitis, encephalitis, Bell's palsy, esophagitis (especially in HIV), disseminated disease.
- Recurrent episodes preceded prodomal period with pain.

## Diagnosis

- History, physical exam.
- Direct fluorescent antibodies or viral cultures confirm the diagnosis.

## Management
### *Primary HSV*

- Acyclovir (Zovirax), 400 mg PO tid × 7–10 d or 200 mg PO 5×/d × 7–10 d
- Famciclovir (Famvir), 250 mg PO tid × 7–10 d
- Valacyclovir (Valtrex), 1 g PO bid × 7–10 d

### *Recurrent HSV*

- Reduces severity and duration of recurrent episodes
- Acyclovir, 400 mg PO tid × 5 d or 200 mg 5×/d × 5 d
- Famciclovir, 125 mg PO bid × 5 d

- Valacyclovir, 500 mg PO bid × 3–5 d or 1 g PO × 5 d

### *Suppressive Therapy*

- If >6 recurrences/yr
- Acyclovir, 400 mg PO bid
- Famciclovir, 250 mg PO bid
- Valacyclovir, 250 mg PO bid or 1 g PO qd

## CHANCROID

- *Haemophilus ducreyi*
- Painful, nonindurated genital ulcers with undermined edges
- Inguinal adenopathy often present

### Diagnosis

Inguinal lymph node biopsy with small, pleomorphic gram-negative bacilli

### Management

- Ceftriaxone (Rocephin), 250 mg IM × 1
- Erythromycin (E-Mycin, EES, Ery-Tab, Eryc, EryPed, Ilosone), 500 mg PO qid × 7 d
- Azithromycin, 1 g PO × 1
- Ciprofloxacin (Cipro, Cipro XR), 500 mg PO bid × 3 d

## LYMPHOGRANULOMA VENERUM

- *Chlamydia trachomatis*
- Primary infection: painless vulvar ulcer
- Secondary phase: inguinal lymphadenopathy, painful and matted lymph nodes

### Diagnosis

Culture of pus or serum antibody titers

### Management

- Doxycycline, 100 mg PO bid × 21 d
- Erythromycin base, 500 mg PO qid × 21 d (alternate)

## GRANULOMA INGUINALE

- *Calymmatobacterium granulomatis*

- Nodules that ulcerate and bleed

## Diagnosis

Donovan bodies on smear

## Management

- Doxycycline, 100 mg PO bid × 21 d
- TMP-SMX (Bactrim DS), 1 PO bid × 21 d

## CONDYLOMATA ACUMINATA

- HPV
- Verrucous papules
- Spontaneous remissions and recurrences

## Diagnosis

Inspection

## Management

### Patient-Applied Therapy

- Podofilox (Condylox) 0.5%, bid × 3 d (unknown pregnancy safety)
- Imiquimod (Aldara) 5%, 3×/wk × 16 wks (unknown pregnancy safety)

### Clinician-Applied Therapy

- Podophyllin 10–25%, every week (unknown pregnancy safety)
- Trichloroacetic acid weekly
- Cryotherapy
- Laser therapy

## MOLLUSCUM CONTAGIOSUM

- Poxvirus
- Flesh-colored, dome-shaped papules with central umbilication

## Diagnosis

Inspection

## Management

- Usually self-limited
- Mechanical destruction by curettage, cryotherapy, laser used for cosmesis

- Cantharidin (blistering agent) also used

## PEDICULOSIS PUBIS

- *Phthirus pubis* (louse)
- Inflammation, vulvar pruritus

### Diagnosis

Visualization of lice; microscopic exam with mineral oil

### Management

- Lindane (Kwell) 1% shampoo × 4 mins (not recommended in pregnancy)
- Permethrin (Elimite, Nix) 1% cream for 10 mins
- Pyrethrins with piperonyl butoxide × 10 mins
- Launder clothes in hot water
- Treat sexual partners

## SCABIES

- *Sarcoptes scabiei* (parasite)
- Transmission: contact
- Pruritus over entire body
- Papules and burrows may be visualized

### Diagnosis

Inspection, microscopy

### Management

- Permethrin 5% cream over entire body, wash off in 8–14 hrs
- Lindane 1% lotion over entire body, wash off in 8 hrs (alternate)
- Ivermectin (Stromectol), 200 µg/kg PO repeat in 2 wks
- Launder in hot water, dry all clothes, linens
- Treat sexual partners

## REFERENCE

1. Centers for Disease Control and Prevention: 2002 Guidelines for treatment of sexually transmitted diseases. *MMWR Morb Mortal Wkly Rep* 2002;51:1–80.

# Contraception

# 57

# Oral Contraceptive Pills

*Management of oral contraceptive pills (OCPs)*

## INTRODUCTION
Failure rate: perfect use (0.1%), typical use (3.0%)

## PHARMACOLOGY
- Include an estrogen and progestin
- Mechanism: inhibit gonadotropin secretion
- Estrogen: ethinyl estradiol is major estrogen
- Estrogen suppresses FSH, prevents follicular development
- Progestin: from 19-nortestosterone family
  - Desogestrel, gestodene, norgestimate
- Progestin inhibits LH release, suppresses ovulation, causes endometrial decidualization, thickened cervical mucus, decreased tubal peristalsis
- See Table 57-1

## MEDICAL COMPLICATIONS
### Venous Thromboembolism
- Increased risk related to the estrogenic component.
- Relative risk three- to fourfold higher than general population for low-dose OCPs [1].
- Screen family or personal history of thromboembolic phenomenon for hereditary thrombophilia.

### Myocardial Infarction and Stroke
- No increased risk for <35-year-old nonsmoker on low-dose OCPs.
- HTN, older age, tobacco use are risk factors [2].
- OCPs contraindicated in smokers aged >35.

### Lipoproteins
Progestin component increases LDL, decreases HDL.

**TABLE 57-1.**
**DEFINITIONS OF AVAILABLE ORAL CONTRACEPTIVE**
**PILL PREPARATIONS**

Low dose: contain <50 μg of ethinyl estradiol

First generation (high dose): contain >50 μg of ethinyl estradiol

Second generation: contain levonorgestrel, norgestimate, and other members of the norethindrone family and 30 or 35 μg of ethinyl estradiol

Third generation: contains desogestrel or gestodene with 20 or 30 μg of ethinyl estradiol

Monophasic formulations: contain the same amount of hormone in each tablet.

Triphasic formulations: contain variable amounts of estrogen and progestin in the active pills.

### Cholelithiasis

Estrogen causes slight increase in cholelithiasis in first year of OCP use.

### Cancer

- Protective against endometrial and ovarian cancer [3].
- High-dose OCPs increase the risk of breast cancer (relative risk of current users is 1.24) and liver adenomas [4].

### Future Fertility

- May take several months for fertility to return after cessation of OCP use
- No long-term fertility effects

### Hypertension

- Associated with the use of high-dose OCPs
- Effects reversible 36 mos after discontinuation

### CONTRAINDICATIONS

- See Table 57-2.
- Low-dose OCPs may be considered in stable diabetes, HTN, and seizure disorder.

### CLINICAL CONSIDERATIONS
### Menstrual Irregularities

- Breakthrough bleeding: secondary to endometrial decidualization

**TABLE 57-2.**
**CONTRAINDICATIONS TO ORAL CONTRACEPTIVE PILL USE**

| Absolute | Relative |
|---|---|
| History or family history of venous thromboembolism | Migraine headache with aura |
| | HTN |
| Thrombophlebitis | Prolonged diabetes mellitus |
| Impaired liver function | Anticonvulsant medications |
|    Hepatic adenoma, carcinoma | SLE |
|    Jaundice, cholestasis, hepatitis | Hypertriglyceridemia (>350 mg/dL ) |
| Breast cancer | |
| Undiagnosed vaginal bleeding | Sickle cell disease |
| Pregnancy | Undergoing surgery |
| Smokers aged >35 | |
| Previous MI or stroke | |
| Significant cardiovascular disease | |

- Rule out pregnancy
- Prescribe 3- to 7-d course of CEE (1.25 mg PO qd) or estradiol (2 mg PO qd)
- OCP with higher dose of estrogen
- Amenorrhea: small fraction of OCP users secondary endometrial decidualization
  - Rule out pregnancy
  - Reassurance

## Acne

OCPs increase sex hormone–binding globulin and improve acne

## Drug Interactions

- Certain anticonvulsants and antibiotics induce hepatic clearance of OCPs
- Avoid OCPs in patients receiving:
  - Phenobarbital
  - Carbamazepine

**TABLE 57-3.**
**RECOMMENDATIONS FOR MISSED PILLS**

| Pills missed | Recommendation | Backup contraception |
|---|---|---|
| 1 | Take pill as soon as possible | None |
| 2 (wks 1 or 2) | Take 2 pills daily for 2 d | Yes (7 d) |
| 2 (wk 3) or ≥3 | Day 1 start: start new pill pack | Yes (7 d) |
| | Sunday start: take pill daily until Sunday, then start new pack | |

- Felbamate
- Rifampin
- Phenytoin
- Primidone
- Topiramate
- Griseofulvin

### Future Fertility

- May take several months for fertility to return after cessation of OCPs.
- No long-term fertility effect.

### Missed Pills

See Table 57-3.

### Other Side Effects

- Emotional lability
- Nausea
- Weight gain (5–7 lbs)
- Breast discomfort
- Headaches

### PROGESTIN-ONLY PILL

- OCP formulation taken every day without hormone-free interval
- Progestin content is lower than standard combination OCPs

### Pharmacology

- Thickens cervical mucus, causes endometrial decidualization.

- Ovulation still occurs in 40% of cycles.

- Effects of pill last only 24 hrs: must take at same time every day.

- Started on first day of menses and backup method used for 7 d.

## Clinical Considerations

- Option for women in whom combination OCPs are contraindicated because of the estrogen content

- Does not inhibit milk production: good choice for lactating women

## SUGGESTED READING

American College of Obstetricians and Gynecologists. *The use of hormonal contraception in women with coexisting medical conditions. ACOG Practice Bulletin 18.* Washington, DC: ACOG, 2000.

Speroff L, Glass RH, Kase NG. *Clinical gynecologic endocrinology and infertility*, 6th ed. Philadelphia: Lippincott Williams & Wilkins, 1999.

## REFERENCES

1. WHO Collaborative Study of Cardiovascular Disease and Steroid Hormone Contraception. Venous thromboembolic disease and combined oral contraceptives: results of international multicentre case-control study. *Lancet* 1995;348:1582.

2. WHO Collaborative Study of Cardiovascular Disease and Steroid Hormone Contraception. Acute myocardial infarction and combined oral contraceptives: results of an international multicentre case-control study. *Lancet* 1997;349:1202.

3. The Cancer and Steroid Hormone Study of the CDC and NICHD. The reduction in risk of ovarian cancer associated with oral contraceptive use. *N Engl J Med* 1987;316:650.

4. Collaborative Group on Hormonal Factors in Breast Cancer. Breast cancer and hormonal contraceptives: collaborative reanalysis of individual data on 53,297 women with breast cancer and 100,239 women without breast cancer from 54 epidemiological studies. *Lancet* 1996;347:1713.

# 58 Emergency Contraception

*A prescription for emergency contraception may be provided to patients*

## INTRODUCTION

Patients may be given a prescription for emergency contraception at a routine office visit so that it is available if the need arises. All women requesting emergency contraception should be counseled about long-term methods of contraception and sexual disease transmission.

## COMBINED ORAL CONTRACEPTIVE PILLS (YUZPE METHOD)

- Two large doses of combined estrogen and progestin oral contraceptive pills [1]
- First dose taken within 72 hrs of unprotected intercourse for maximum effect
- Second dose taken 12 hrs later
- Efficacy: 75%
- Antiemetic prescribed for nausea, e.g., compazine 10 mg PO q6
- See Table 58-1

## PROGESTIN-ONLY PILLS

- Two doses of progestin-only pills taken 12 hrs apart.
- First dose taken within 72 hrs of unprotected intercourse.
- Efficacy: 65–85%.
- See Table 58-2.

## COPPER INTRAUTERINE DEVICE

- Inserted up to 5 d after ovulation to prevent unwanted pregnancy
- Efficacy: 99%

## TABLE 58-1.
## COMBINED ORAL EMERGENCY
## CONTRACEPTIVE REGIMENS

Preven: Prepackaged kit designed for emergency contraception. 100 µg ethinyl estradiol and 0.50 mg levonorgestrel. Two + two pills 12 hrs apart.

Two + two pills 12 hrs apart

**Ovral:** 0.05 mg ethinyl estradiol/0.50 mg norgestrel

Four +four pills 12 hrs apart

**Lo-Ovral:** 0.30 mg of norgestrel/0.03 µg ethinyl estradiol

**Levora:** 0.15 mg levonorgestrel/30 µg ethinyl estradiol

**Levlen 28:** 0.15 mg levonorgestrel/30 µg ethinyl estradiol

**Nordette 28:** 0.15 mg levonorgestrel/30 µg ethinyl estradiol

**Triphasil:** 0.125 mg levonorgestrel/30 µg ethinyl estradiol

**Trilevlen:** 0.125 mg levonorgestrel/30 µg ethinyl estradiol

**Trivora:** 0.050 mg levonorgestrel/30 µg ethinyl estradiol

Five + five pills 12 hrs apart

**Alesse:** 0.1 mg levonorgestrel/20 µg ethinyl estradiol

**Levlite:** 0.1 mg levonorgestrel/20 µg ethinyl estradiol

## TABLE 58-2.
## PROGESTIN-ONLY EMERGENCY
## CONTRACEPTION REGIMENS

**Plan B:** Prepackaged kit designed for emergency contraception

0.75 mg levonorgestrel. One + one pill 12 hrs apart.

20 + 20 pills 12 hrs apart

**Ovrette:** (0.075 mg levonorgestrel)

## SUGGESTED READING

Speroff L, Glass RH, Kase NG. *Clinical gynecologic endocrinology and infertility*, 6th ed. Philadelphia: Lippincott Williams & Wilkins, 1999.

## REFERENCE

1. Task Force on Postovulatory Methods of Fertility Regulation. Randomized controlled trial of levonorgestrel versus Yuzpe regimen of combined oral contraceptives for emergency contraception. *Lancet* 1998;352:428–433.

# 59 Barrier Methods of Contraception

*Available barrier methods of contraception*

## CONDOMS

- Failure rate: 14%
- Breakage: 1–8/1000
- Most latex, some silicone, polyurethane, or lamb intestine
- Placed before intercourse; removed after coitus
- Avoid oil-based lubricants

## DIAPHRAGMS

- Failure rate: 18–20%
- Types: arcing spring, coil spring, flat spring, wide seal
- Must be fitted by physician with patient instruction
- Side effects: vaginal irritation, UTI
- Placed not >6 hrs before sex and left in place 6–24 hrs after

## CERVICAL CAPS

- Failure rate: 18–20%.
- Prentif cap comes in four sizes and must be fit by physician.
- Spermicidal gel helps reduce failures.
- Cap removed 8 hrs after coitus.

## FEMALE CONDOMS

- Failure rate: 21%
- Pouch of polyurethane placed into vagina
- Inserted 8 hrs before coitus
- Side effects: UTI

## SPERMICIDES

- Failure rate: 20–25%.
- Used alone or with diaphragms, condoms, cervical caps.

## TABLE 59-1.
## SPERMICIDES

| | |
|---|---|
| Vaginal contraceptive film | VCF (70 mg nonoxynol-9) |
| Foams | Delfen (nonoxynol-9, 12.5%) |
| | Emko (nonoxynol-9, 8%) |
| | Koromex (nonoxynol-9, 12.5%) |
| Jellies and creams | Conceptrol (nonoxynol-9, 4%) |
| | Delfen (nonoxynol-9, 12.5%) |
| | Ortho-Gynol (nonoxynol-9, 3%) |
| | Ramses (nonoxynol-9, 5%) |
| | Koromex jelly (nonoxynol-9, 3%) |
| Suppositories | Encare (nonoxynol-9, 2.27%) |
| | Koromex inserts (nonoxynol-9, 125 mg) |
| | Semicid (nonoxynol-9, 100 mg) |

Reprinted from Speroff L, Glass RH, Kase NG. *Clinical gynecologic endocrinology and infertility*, 6th ed. Philadelphia: Lippincott Williams & Wilkins, 1999:1003–1004, with permission.

- Applied 30 mins before coitus.
- Tablets and suppositories last 1 hr; jellies, creams, and foams 8 hrs.
- See Table 59-1.

# 60

# Long-Acting Methods of Contraception

*Injectables, rods, rings, and patches*

## DEPOT-MEDROXYPROGESTERONE ACETATE (DEPO-PROVERA, DMPA)

- Injectable medroxyprogesterone acetate
- Failure rate 0.3%

### Pharmacology

- Blocks LH surge, thickens cervical mucus, causes endometrial atrophy
- Given within 7 d of menses (or provide backup method)
- Injections given q11–13wks

### Contraindications

See Table 60-1.

### Clinical Problems

- Menstrual bleeding: secondary to endometrial decidualization.
  - 70% in first year, 80% amenorrheic by 5 yrs
  - Treatment: CEE, 1.25 mg; or estradiol, 2 mg × 7 d
- Breast cancer: slight increase risk in first year [1].
- Lipoprotein profile: effects uncertain.
- Future fertility: delay in conception averages 9 mos; no long-term effect.
- Bone density: small decrease may occur with long-term use.
- Other side effects include breast tenderness, weight gain, and depression.

## COMBINED INJECTABLES (LUNELLE)

- Suspension of 25 mg medroxyprogesterone acetate and 5 mg estradiol cypionate.
- Failure rate is 0.1–0.4%.

## TABLE 60-1.
## CONTRAINDICATIONS TO DEPOT-
## MEDROXYPROGESTERONE ACETATE

| Absolute | Relative |
| --- | --- |
| Pregnancy | Liver disease |
| Unexplained vaginal bleeding | Severe cardiovascular disease |
| Coagulation disorders | Rapid return of fertility desired |
| Liver adenoma | Severe depression |

### Pharmacology

- Mechanism similar to OCPs
- Injected q28d

### Contraindications

Similar to those for OCPs

### Clinical Problems

- Depression
- Anxiety
- Weight gain
- Mood lability

### NORPLANT

- Six Silastic rods containing levonorgestrel implanted in upper arm
- Functions 5 yrs
- Failure rate 0.05%

### Pharmacology

- Creates an atrophic endometrium, thickens cervical mucus, one-third of cycles are ovulatory.
- Backup contraception given for the first 3 d of use.

### Contraindications

See Table 60-2.

### Clinical Problems

- Menstrual bleeding: 80% secondary to endometrial decidualization
  - Amenorrhea develops in <10%
  - Treatment: CEE, 1.25 mg; or estradiol, 2 mg × 7 d

**TABLE 60-2.**
**CONTRAINDICATIONS TO NORPLANT**

| Absolute | Relative |
|---|---|
| Thromboembolic disease | Heavy tobacco use |
| Undiagnosed vaginal bleeding | Age >35 yrs |
| Acute liver disease | History of ectopic pregnancy |
| Liver neoplasms | Diabetes mellitus |
| Breast cancer | Hypercholesterolemia |
| Pregnancy | HTN |
| Active thrombophlebitis | Cardiovascular/cerebrovascular disease |
| | Biliary disease |
| | Immunocompromise |

- Ectopic pregnancy: 30% of pregnancies
- Future fertility: return of fertility is prompt; no long-term effects
- Other side effects: weight gain, mastalgia, headache, galactorrhea, acne, ovarian cysts

## TRANSDERMAL CONTRACEPTIVE SYSTEM

- Ortho Evra Patch
  - Apply patch for 3 consecutive wks followed by 1 patch-free wk
  - Withdrawal bleed during patch-free week
- Efficacy similar to OCPs
- Backup contraception or new patch required if patch removed for >24 hours during 3-wk period
- Avoid if weight >90 kg (198 lbs)

## VAGINAL RING

- NuvaRing
- Inserted and worn for 3 consecutive wks followed by 1 ring-free wk
  - Withdrawal bleeding during ring-free week
- Backup contraception if ring removed for >3 hrs

## REFERENCE

1. WHO Collaborative Study of Neoplasia and Steroid Contraceptives. Breast cancer and depot-medroxyprogesterone acetate: a multinational study. *Lancet* 1991;338:833.

# 61 Intrauterine Device

*Management of the intrauterine device (IUD)*

## PHARMACOLOGY

- Copper IUD: sterile inflammation that is spermicidal, prevents implantation
  - Approved for 10 yrs
- Levonorgestrel IUD: inflammation, endometrial decidualization
  - Approved for 10 yrs
- Progestasert: inflammation, cervical mucus thickening
  - Approved for 1 yr
  - Lower bleeding than copper
  - Failure rate: 0.1–2%

## CONTRAINDICATIONS

See Table 61-1.

## INSERTION

- Best inserted after menses
- NSAID may be administered
- Cervix is visualized, prepared with antiseptic solution, grasped with tenaculum
- Paracervical block may be administered
- Uterine cavity sounded, loaded IUD placed
- String cut to 4 cm from os; patient taught to palpate string
- Antibiotic prophylaxis not needed

## CLINICAL PROBLEMS

- Infection: pelvic infection increased first month after insertion [2]
- Severe infection requires IUD removal
- *Actinomyces* infection: ampicillin (250 mg qid × 14 d), IUD removal
- Displaced string: locate IUD by U/S, radiography, or hysteroscopy

## TABLE 61-1.
## CONTRAINDICATIONS TO IUD

| Absolute | Relative |
|----------|----------|
| Pregnancy | Abnormal uterine cavity |
| Pelvic malignancy | Immunosuppression |
| Undiagnosed vaginal bleeding | Nulligravidity |
| Pelvic infection | Abnormal Pap smear |
| High-risk STD behavior | History of ectopic pregnancy |
| Wilson's disease | |

- Pregnancy: 2–3% will be ectopic
- Intrauterine pregnancy: IUD removed if string visible
- If string not visible, U/S-guided removal can be attempted
    - If IUD left in place, risk of septic abortion and preterm labor is increased
- Future fertility: prompt return of fertility, no long-term consequences

## REFERENCES

1. Speroff L, Glass RH, Kase NG. *Clinical gynecologic endocrinology and infertility*, 6th ed. Philadelphia: Lippincott & Williams & Wilkins, 1999.
2. Farley MM, Rosenberg MJ, Rowe PJ, et al. Intrauterine devices and pelvic inflammatory disease: an international perspective. *Lancet* 1992;339:785.

# 62

# Sterilization

*Permanent methods of surgical sterilization*

## MINILAPAROTOMY

- 2- to 5-cm subumbilical incision (postpartum) or suprapubic (interval bilateral tubal ligation) incision

- Each fallopian tube identified and ligated (methods in Fig. 62-1)

## LAPAROSCOPIC TUBAL LIGATION

- **Bipolar cautery:** Klepinger forceps used to coagulate 2- to 3-cm segment of tube

  - Highest risk of fistula formation

- **Silastic bands** (fallope rings, Yoon band): band applied around knuckle of tube

- **Spring clips** (Hulka-Clemens, Filshie clips): clip applied 1–2 cm distal to the cornu

  - Highest chance of reversibility

## CLINICAL PROBLEMS

- Failure

  - Unipolar coagulation: 0.75%

  - Postpartum excision: 0.75%

  - Silastic rings: 1.77%

  - Interval excision: 2.01%

  - Bipolar cautery: 2.48%

  - Spring clip: 3.65%

- Ectopic pregnancy increased if bilateral tubal ligation failure [1]

- **Menstrual function:** long-term effects uncertain

- **Reversibility:** results best when only small segment of tube damaged

- **Other effects:** protective against PID, may be protective against ovarian cancer

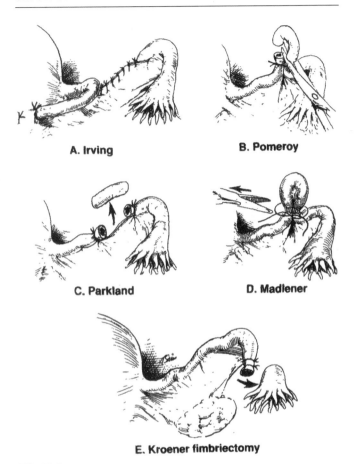

**A. Irving**

**B. Pomeroy**

**C. Parkland**

**D. Madlener**

**E. Kroener fimbriectomy**

**FIG. 62-1.**
Methods of sterilization by minilaparotomy. (Reprinted from Cunningham FG, MacDonald PC, Gant NF, et al. *Williams obstetrics*, 21st ed. McGraw-Hill, 2001:1556, with permission.)

## SUGGESTED READING

Cunningham FG, MacDonald PC, Gant NF, et al. *Williams obstetrics*, 20th ed. Appleton & Lange, 1997.

## REFERENCE

1. Peterson HB, Xia Z, Hughes JM, et al. The risk of pregnancy after tubal sterilization: findings from the U.S. Collaborative Review of Sterilization. *Am J Obstet Gynecol* 1996;174:1161–1170.

# Urogynecology

# 63 Urinary Incontinence

*Urinary incontinence often goes unrecognized*

## DIFFERENTIAL DIAGNOSIS
See Table 63-1.

## HISTORY
- Urine loss: when, how often, how much, provocations, treatments
- Medical history: DM, vascular disease, neurologic disease
- Medications

## PHYSICAL EXAM
- Exam while laying and standing with provocation by coughing
- Pelvic exam for prolapse
- Neurologic exam

## DIAGNOSTIC EVALUATION
- UA with culture and cytology
- Postvoid residual
- Frequency/volume chart: record time, amount, and associated activity with incontinence
  - Normal values: 7–8 voids/day, 1500–2500 mL/day urine, largest void 400–600 mL, average void 250 mL
  - Optional studies: cystoscopy, urethroscopy

## URODYNAMICS
### Subtracted cystometry
- Measures intravesical pressure and intraabdominal pressure to determine detrusor pressure
- Bladder filled and provocation with coughing performed
- Stress incontinence: urine loss with provocation
- Detrusor overactivity: detrusor contractions result in urine loss without provocation

### TABLE 63-1.
### DIFFERENTIAL DIAGNOSIS OF URINARY INCONTINENCE

| Transurethral | Extraurethral |
|---|---|
| Genuine stress incontinence | Congenital |
|    Bladder neck displacement |    Ectopic ureter |
|    Intrinsic sphincteric deficiency |    Bladder exstrophy |
|    Combined |    Other |
| Detrusor overactivity | Fistulas |
|    Detrusor instability |    Ureteric |
|    Detrusor hyperreflexia |    Vesical |
| Mixed incontinence |    Urethral |
| Urinary retention with overflow |    Complex |
| Urethral diverticulum | |
| Congenital urethral abnormalities | |
| Functional and transient incontinence | |

Reprinted from Berek JS, Adashi EY, Hillard PA. *Novak's gynecology*, 12th ed. Philadelphia: Williams & Wilkins 1996:630, with permission.

### Leak-Point Pressure

Intravesical pressure when stress incontinence occurs

### STRESS URINARY INCONTINENCE

- Occurs when increased intraabdominal pressure raises intravesical pressure above urethral closure pressure with urine loss
- Etiology: bladder neck displacement or intrinsic sphincteric deficiency

### Diagnosis

- Incontinence when intraabdominal pressure increased
- Urodynamics described above

### Management

- Initial treatment: muscle-strengthening exercises (30% cured).
- If muscle strengthening fails: surgical management may be undertaken [1].
- Treat detrusor overactivity before surgery if mixed incontinence.
- See Table 63-2.

## TABLE 63-2.
## MANAGEMENT OF STRESS URINARY INCONTINENCE

| Treatment | Comment |
| --- | --- |
| Muscle-strengthening (Kegel) exercises | Contracting muscles of pelvic floor. |
| | Perform for 5 secs, 15–20×/day. |
| | Must be properly instructed. |
| | May be facilitated by use of weighted vaginal cones. |
| Estrogen therapy | All postmenopausal patients with stress urinary incontinence be placed on estrogen (HRT). |
| Electrical stimulation | Electrical stimulation of pelvic floor musculature. |
| Anterior colporrhaphy | Should be used only for cystocele repair. |
| | Poor long-term success for stress urinary incontinence. |
| Retropubic urethropexy | Surgical treatment of choice for bladder neck displacement. |
| Marshall-Marchetti-Krantz (MMK) procedure | Periurethral fascia attached to pubic symphysis. |
| | Osteitis pubis may complicate. |
| Burch colposuspension | Bladder neck fascia attached to iliopectineal ligament. |
| Needle suspension (Pereyra procedure) | Suture placed from abdominal incision to endopelvic. |
| | Fascia at the level of the bladder neck. |
| | Lower 5-yr success rate than Burch or MMK. |
| Sling procedures (transvaginal taping, TVT) | Treatment of choice for intrinsic sphincteric deficiency. |
| Periurethral injections | Treatment for intrinsic sphincteric deficiency. Collagen injected periurethrally. |

## DETRUSOR OVERACTIVITY

- Unintentional detrusor contractions result in incontinence
- Detrusor hyperreflexia if neurologic disorder, detrusor instability if no neurologic abnormality

### Diagnosis

- Episodes of incontinence any time
- Urodynamic findings described above

**TABLE 63-3.**
## TREATMENT OF DETRUSOR OVERACTIVITY

| Treatment | Comments |
|---|---|
| Timed voidings | Start at frequent intervals (hourly) |
| | Patient should void whether she has to or not |
| | After 1 successful wk, increase voiding schedule by 15-min intervals |
| Drug therapy | Propantheline bromide (Pro-Banthine), 15–30 mg PO qid |
| | Hyoscyamine sulfate (Levsin), 0.125–0.25 mg PO q4–6h |
| | Hyoscyamine sulfate extended release (Levsin), 0.375 mg PO bid |
| | Oxybutynin chloride (Ditropan), 5–10 mg PO tid–qid |
| | Dicyclomine hydrochloride (Bentyl), 20 mg PO qid |
| | Tolterodine (Detrol), 1–2 mg PO bid |

### Management

- Initial treatment: timed voidings.
- If timed voidings fail: pharmacotherapy.
- See Table 63-3.

### FUNCTIONAL (TRANSIENT) INCONTINENCE

Reversible causes of incontinence: delirium, infection, atrophic vaginitis, drugs (sedatives, anticholinergics, alpha antagonists), psychological, excessive urine production, restricted mobility, fecal impaction

### SUGGESTED READING

Berek JS, Adashi EY, Hillard PA. *Novak's gynecology*, 12th ed. Philadelphia: Williams & Wilkins, 1996.

### REFERENCE

1. Bergman A, Ballard CA, Kooning PP. Comparision of three different surgical procedures for genuine stress incontinence: prospective randomized study. *Am J Obstet Gynecol* 1989;160:1102–1106.

# 64 Pelvic Organ Prolapse

*Pelvic organ prolapse is common and often unrecognized in the elderly*

## EVALUATION

- Pelvic organ prolapse is now described based on reference points A–D (Fig. 64-1).
- The degree of prolapse is graded in centimeters above (negative) or below (positive) the hymen.

## CYSTOCELE

Anterior vaginal wall prolapse results in acystocele or urethrocele.

### History

- Urgency
- Frequency
- Incontinence
- Incomplete bladder emptying
- Pelvic pressure

### Physical Exam

- One blade of speculum placed against posterior vaginal wall: anterior wall bulge when bearing down
- Exclude infected Skene's gland or urethral diverticula

### Management

- Nonoperative interventions: Kegel exercises, estrogen replacement, pessary
- Surgical: anterior colporrhapy (repair rectocele if also present)

## RECTOCELE

Posterior vaginal wall prolapse results in rectocele

### History

- Constipation
- Difficulty in defecating
- Support vaginal wall to defecate
- Pressure

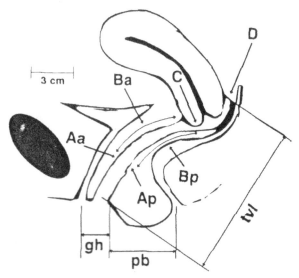

**FIG. 64-1.**
Terminology of pelvic organ prolapse.

## Physical Exam

One blade of speculum placed against anterior vaginal wall: posterior wall bulge when bearing down

## Management

- Nonoperative interventions: Kegel exercises, estrogen replacement, pessary

- Surgical: posterior colporrhapy and perineorrhaphy (repair cystocele if also present)

## ENTEROCELE

- Herniation of small bowel.

- Most commonly enteroceles involve posterior vaginal wall near vaginal fornix.

## History

- Pelvic pressure

- Heaviness

- Sense that "something is falling out"

## Physical Exam

- Bulge where enterocele located (usually posterior vaginal wall)
- Contents of herniation sometimes reducible

## Management

- Usually surgical
- Transvaginal enterocele repair: enterocele incised, contents reduced, and enterocele sac ligated with purse-string suture

## UTERINE PROLAPSE

- Uterus and cervix protrude downward into vagina.
- Complete uterine prolapse is known as uterine procidentia.
- Graded based on degree of descent.

## History

- Pelvic pressure
- Heaviness
- Sense that "something is falling out"

## Physical Exam

- Visualize uterine descent.
- Identify any ulcerated areas.

## Management

- Nonoperative interventions: Kegel exercises, estrogen replacement, pessary
- Surgical: vaginal hysterectomy, colpocleisis if no longer sexually active

## VAGINAL VAULT PROLAPSE

Vaginal vault (posthysterectomy) prolapse: vaginal cuff descends into vagina

## History

- Pelvic pressure
- Heaviness
- Sense that "something is falling out"

## Physical Exam

Visualize vaginal vault descent.

## Management

- Nonoperative: pessary (often unsuccessful)
- Surgical: sacrospinous ligament fixation or sacral colpopexy

## SUGGESTED READING

Berek JS, Adashi EY, Hillard PA. *Novak's gynecology*, 12th ed. Philadelphia: Williams & Wilkins, 1996.

Bump RC, Mattiasson A, Bo K, et al. The standardization of terminology of female pelvic organ prolapse and pelvic floor dysfunction. *Am J Obstet Gynecol* 1996;175:10–17.

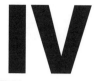

# IV

# Reproductive Endocrinology

# 65 | **Menstrual Cycle**

*Endocrine changes during the menstrual cycle*

Fig. 65-1 depicts the menstrual cycle.

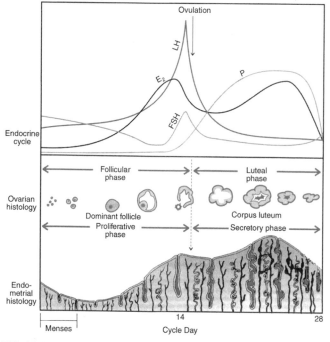

**FIG. 65-1.**
Menstrual cycle. (Reprinted from Berek JS, Adashi EY, Hillard PA. *Novak's gynecology*, 12th ed. Philadelphia: Williams & Wilkins, 1996:160, with permission.)

## SUGGESTED READING

Berek JS, Adashi EY, Hillard PA. *Novak's gynecology*, 12th ed. Philadelphia: Williams & Wilkins, 1996.

# Puberty

*Pubertal development follows a normal sequence of events*

## PHYSIOLOGY

- At puberty, pulsatile GnRH secretion develops.
- Average age at onset of puberty: 8–9 (black), 10 (white).
- Puberty follows a normal sequence (Table 66-1).

## PRECOCIOUS PUBERTY

Pubertal development before age 8.

### Differential Diagnosis

- Idiopathic precocious puberty is diagnosis of exclusion (Table 66-2).
- McCune-Albright syndrome (polyostotic fibrous dysplasia): multiple cystic osseous lesions, café au lait spots, precocious puberty.
- Suspect CNS lesion in patients aged <4.

### Diagnostic Evaluation

- History
- Rapid pubertal development heightens possibility of neoplastic process

### Physical Exam

- Height, weight, growth records
- Breast, genital development (Tanner stages), and signs of hirsuitism
- Abdominal and pelvic exams
- Neurologic exam

### Lab Evaluation

- FSH, LH, hCG, TSH
- GnRH challenge (100 µg GnRH, LH 40 mins later should be <8 IU/L)
- Steroids (dehydroepiandrosterone, testosterone, 17 hydroxy-progesterone, estradiol)

## TABLE 66-1.
## SEQUENCE OF NORMAL PUBERTAL DEVELOPMENT

| Milestone | Average age (yrs) |
|---|---|
| Breast bud | 10.5 |
| Onset of pubic hair | 11.0 |
| Maximal growth | 11.4 |
| Menarche | 12.8 |
| Adult breast | 14.6 |
| Adult pubic hair | 13.7 |

## TABLE 66-2.
## DIFFERENTIAL DIAGNOSIS OF PRECOCIOUS PUBERTY

| | Girls (%) | Boys (%) |
|---|---|---|
| GnRH dependent (true precocity) | | |
|   Idiopathic | 74.0 | 41.0 |
|   CNS disease | 7.0 | 26.0 |
|     Infections (meningitis, encephalitis) | | |
|     Neoplasms (craniopharyngioma, hamartoma, astrocytoma, glioma, neurofibroma, pineal tumor) | | |
|   Hydrocephalus | | |
|   von Recklinghausen's disease | | |
| Trauma | | |
|   GnRH independent (precocious pseudopuberty) | | |
|   Ovarian (cyst or neoplasm) | 11.0 | — |
|   Testicular | — | 10.0 |
|   McCune-Albright syndrome | 5.0 | 1.0 |
|   Adrenal feminizing | 1.0 | 0 |
|   Adrenal masculinizing | 1.0 | 22.0 |
|   Ectopic gonadotropin production | 0.5 | 0.5 |
|     Neoplasms (hepatoma, dysgerminoma, chorioepithelioma) | | |

Reprinted from Speroff L, Glass RH, Kase NG. *Clinical gynecologic endocrinology and infertility*, 6th ed. Philadelphia: Lippincott Williams & Wilkins, 1999:393, with permission.

**TABLE 66-3.**
**DIFFERENTIAL DIAGNOSIS OF DELAYED PUBERTY**

|  | Frequency (%) |
|---|---|
| Hypergonadotropic hypogonadism | 43.0 |
|   Ovarian failure/abnormal karyotype | 26.0 |
|   Ovarian failure/normal karyotype | 17.0 |
|     46 XX | 15.0 |
|     46 XY | 2.0 |
| Hypogonadotropic hypogonadism | 31.0 |
|   Reversible | 18.0 |
|     Physiologic delay | 10.0 |
|     Weight loss/anorexia | 3.0 |
|     Primary hypothyroidism | 1.0 |
|     Congenital adrenal hyperplasia | 1.0 |
|     Cushing syndrome | 0.5 |
|     Prolactinoma | 1.5 |
|   Irreversible | 13.0 |
| GnRH deficiency | 7.0 |
|     Hypopituitarism | 2.0 |
|     Congenital CNS defect | 0.5 |
|     Other pituitary adenoma | 0.5 |
|     Craniopharyngioma | 1.0 |
|     Malignant pituitary tumor | 0.5 |
| Eugonadism | 26.0 |
|   Müllerian agenesis | 14.0 |
|   Vaginal septum | 3.0 |
|   Imperforate hymen | 0.5 |
|   Androgen insensitivity syndrome | 1.0 |
|   Inappropriate positive feedback | 7.0 |

Reprinted from Speroff L, Glass RH, Kase NG. *Clinical gynecologic endocrinology and infertility*, 6th ed. Philadelphia: Lippincott Williams & Wilkins, 1999:405, with permission.

## Radiologic Evaluation

- CT/MRI (rule out CNS pathology)
- Bone age (x-ray of wrist)

## Management

- GnRH-dependent precocious puberty: GnRH agonist to suppress gonadotropin secretion.

- Goal of treatment is to maintain estradiol level <10 pg/mL (to maximize adult height).

## DELAYED PUBERTY

- Failure to develop any secondary sexual characteristics by age 13 or absence of menarche by age 16.

- Evaluation probably appropriate if no signs of puberty by age 17.

- Evaluation and treatment are similar to amenorrhea.

### Differential Diagnosis

- See Table 66-3.

### Management

Hormonal therapy can sustain maturation of secondary sexual characteristics, allow achievement of height, and increase bone density.

- CEE, 0.3 mg × 6 mos–1 yr, then CEE, 0.625 mg qd with medroxyprogesterone × 14 d each month

### SUGGESTED READING

Berek JS, Adashi EY, Hillard PA. *Novak's gynecology*, 12th ed. Philadelphia: Williams & Wilkins, 1996.

Speroff L, Glass RH, Kase NG. *Clinical gynecologic endocrinology and infertility*, 6th ed. Philadelphia: Lippincott Williams & Wilkins, 1999.

# 67

# Amenorrhea

*Diagnosis and management of amenorrhea*

## INTRODUCTION

- **Primary** amenorrhea: failure to menstruate by age 16 with secondary sexual characteristics or failure to menstruate by age 14 with absence of secondary sexual characteristics.

- **Secondary** amenorrhea: absence of menses for 6 mos or 3 consecutive menstrual cycles following spontaneous menses.

## Diagnostic Evaluation

### Initial Evaluation

- See Fig. 67-1.

- TSH

  - Elevated: hypothyroidism

- Prolactin

  - Elevated: hyperprolactinemia

- Progestin challenge: 5–10 mg medroxyprogesterone acetate × 10 d

  - If withdrawal bleeding occurs, the etiology of amenorrhea is anovulation

## Follow Up 1

- If withdrawal bleeding does not occur, either the endometrium is not adequately primed or an anatomic anomaly is present.

- Estrogen (2 mg estradiol × 21 d) and a progestin (medroxyprogesterone acetate 5 mg × 10 d) given to attempt withdrawal bleeding.

  - Withdrawal bleeding absent: anatomic problem

## Follow Up 2

- FSH (normal 5–20 IU/L), LH (normal 5–20 IU/L)

  - Low or normal FSH, LH: hypogonadotropic hypogonadism (anterior pituitary or hypothalamus)

- Evaluate with MRI

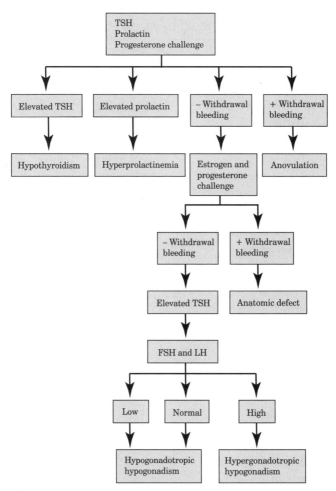

**FIG. 67-1.**
Evaluation of amenorrhea. (Modified from Speroff L, Glass RH, Kase NG. *Clinical gynecologic endocrinology and infertility*, 6th ed. Philadelphia: Lippincott Williams & Wilkins, 1999, p 433.)

- High FSH, LH: hypergonadotropic hypogonadism (ovary)

**Differential Diagnosis**

See Table 67-1.

**TABLE 67-1.**
**DIFFERENTIAL DIAGNOSIS OF AMENORRHEA**

| | |
|---|---|
| Hypothalamic disorders | Ovarian disorders |
|    Hypothyroidism |    Gonadal dysgenesis |
|    Exercise |    Chemotherapy |
|    Anorexia/bulimia |    Radiation |
|    Weight loss |    Infections (mumps) |
|    Stress |    Galactosemia |
|    Anovulation |    Savage syndrome |
|    Chronic diseases |    Autoimmune disease |
|    Craniopharyngioma |    Iatrogenic |
|    Kallman's syndrome | Uterine/outflow tract disorders |
|    Postpill amenorrhea |    Müllerian agenesis |
| Anterior pituitary disorders |    Asherman's syndrome |
|    Pituitary adenomas |    Androgen insensitivity |
|    Empty sella syndrome |    Müllerian anomalies |
|    Lymphocytic hypophysitis |    True hermaphrodites |
|    Sheehan's syndrome | |
|    TB | |
|    Sarcoidosis | |
|    Carotid artery aneurysm | |
|    Dermoid cyst | |
|    Pituitary ablation | |

## Hypothalamic Disorders

- Amenorrhea from lack of GnRH secretion.

- Prolonged hypothalamic amenorrhea requires hormone replacement therapy.

- Kallman's syndrome: amenorrhea and anosmia.

- Postpill amenorrhea: common after hormonal contraception.

  - 6 mos after oral contraceptive pills; 1 yr after depomedroxyprogesterone acetate.

## Anterior Pituitary Disorders

- Pituitary adenomas: prolactinomas most common

- Sheehan's syndrome: pituitary infarction secondary to postpartum hemorrhage

- Lymphocytic hypophysitis: inflammation of the pituitary

## Ovarian Disorders

- Ovarian failure: common after pelvic irradiation or chemotherapy

- Gonadal dysgenesis: absent ovarian function in the presence of abnormal sex chromosomes

  - Etiologies: Turner syndrome (45 XO), mosaics, deletions in X chromosome

  - Karyotype obtained to evaluate chromosomes

  - Male gonad requires gonadectomy to prevent neoplastic transformation

- Savage syndrome: dysfunctional FSH receptors on ovarian follicles

- Idiopathic ovarian failure: ovarian failure before age 40

## Uterine/Outflow Tract Disorders

- Müllerian agenesis (Mayer-Rokitansky-Kuster-Hauser syndrome): faulty müllerian development

  - Vagina, uterus, fallopian tubes absent

  - Renal anomalies common (25%) (should undergo CT and IV pyelogram)

- Asherman's syndrome: multiple intrauterine synechiae after uterine curettage or infection

  - Diagnosis: hysteroscopy or hysterosalpingogram

  - Treatment: hysteroscopic adhesiolysis, estrogen

- Androgen insensitivity (testicular feminization): end-organ resistance to testosterone

  - Karyotype: XY

  - Blind-end vagina present, uterus absent

  - Testes are present, removed after puberty (prevent gonadal tumor)

## MANAGEMENT

- Depends on specific etiology

- Chronic amenorrhea: place on estrogen replacement therapy to prevent bone loss and vaginal atrophy

- Estrogen (0.625 mg CEE or 1 mg estradiol qd) and progesterone (MPA 5 mg × 2 wks each month).

- Oral contraceptive pills are also appropriate.

- Desire pregnancy: ovulation induction

## SUGGESTED READING

Speroff L, Glass RH, Kase NG. *Clinical gynecologic endocrinology and infertility*, 6th ed. Philadelphia: Lippincott Williams & Wilkins, 1999.

Stenchever MA, Droegemueller W, Herbst AL, Mishell DR. *Comprehensive gynecology*. St. Louis: Mosby, 2001.

# 68

# Hirsutism

*Hirsutism is common and often unrecognized in women*

## INTRODUCTION

- Hirsutism: excess hair growth from androgen stimulation
- Virilization: more severe form of hirsutism with accompanying clitoromegaly, male-type pubic hair, temporal balding, deepening voice

## PHYSIOLOGY

- Androgens are derived from ovary and adrenal gland.
- Adrenal gland secretes dehydroepiandrosterone (DHA), dehydroepiandrosterone sulfate (DHAS), testosterone.
- Ovary secretes androstenedione, DHA, testosterone.
- DHA, dehydroepiandrosterone, and androstenedione converted peripherally to testosterone.
- Androgens circulate bound to proteins including sex hormone–binding globulin (SHBG).

### Differential Diagnosis

- Hirsutism results from elevated level of free androgen.
- May result from increased production, exogenous administration, decreased metabolism, or decreased SHBG.
- See Table 68-1.

### Pregnancy

- Results in androgen excess
- Luteoma: solid ovarian enlargment
- Hyperreactio luteinalis: bilateral ovarian cysts
- Both resolve after pregnancy

### Idiopathic Hirsutism

Elevated activity of 5α-reductase, which converts peripheral testosterone to the more active dihydrotestosterone.

## TABLE 68-1.
## DIFFERENTIAL DIAGNOSIS OF HIRSUTISM AND VIRILIZATION

| | |
|---|---|
| Pregnancy | Luteoma |
| | Hyperreactio luteinalis |
| Periphery | Idiopathic hirsutism |
| Ovary | Polycystic ovary syndrome |
| | Stromal hyperthecosis |
| | Ovarian tumor |
| Adrenal gland | Cushing's syndrome |
| | Adrenal tumor |
| | Congenital adrenal hyperplasia |
| Miscellaneous | Exogenous administration |
| | Abnormal gonad/sexual development |

Reprinted from Stenchever MA, Droegemueller W, Herbst AL, Mishell DR. *Comprehensive gynecology*, 4th ed. St. Louis: Mosby, 2001:1148, with permission.

### Ovary

- Polycystic ovary syndrome

- Hyperthecosis: severe form of polycystic ovary syndrome with high levels of testosterone

- Ovarian tumors: Sertoli-Leydig tumors, hilus cell tumors

### Adrenal

- Congenital adrenal hyperplasia: deficiency of 21-hydroxylase, 11β-hydroxylase, or 3β-hydroxysteroid dehydrogenase.

  - Most present during childhood.

  - Late-onset 21-hydroxylase deficiency may escape detection until adulthood.

  - Diagnosis: elevated 17-hydroxyprogesterone.

- Cushing's syndrome: excess glucocorticoid production.

  - Diagnosis: dexamethasone suppression test.

  - Physical findings: buffalo hump, truncal obesity, striae, HTN.

- Adrenal tumors: rare

## Diagnostic Evaluation
### Physical Exam

- Pattern and distribution of hair growth
- Onset of symptoms (rapid onset increases likelihood of malignancy)
- Signs of virilization (clitoromegaly, balding, deepened voice)
- Pelvic exam (adnexal mass)

### Lab Evaluation

- Testosterone, DHA, dexamethasone suppression test
- See Table 68-2.

## MANAGEMENT

Treatment of choice: low-dose oral contraceptive pills

- Reduce ovarian function, elevate SHBG.
- Treatment must be continued for several months until results are apparent.

**TABLE 68-2.**
**LAB EVALUATION OF HIRSUTISM**

| | | |
|---|---|---|
| Testosterone | >200 ng/dL | Pelvic U/S to rule out ovarian tumor |
| | <200 ng/dL | Decreased likelihood of neoplasm |
| DHA | >700 µg/dL | MRI or CT to rule out adrenal neoplasm |
| | 500–700 µg/dL | 17-OHP to rule out late onset CAH |
| | <500 µg/dL | Empiric treatment |
| 17-OHP | >8 ng/dL | Late onset CAH |
| | 2.5–8 ng/dL | ACTH stimulation test to rule out late onset CAH |
| ACTH (cosyntropin) stimulation test | 17-OHP increase >10 ng/dL | Late-onset CAH |
| | 17-OHP increase <10 ng/dL | Late-onset CAH ruled out |
| Low-dose dexamethasone suppression test | Cortisol, >5 mg/dL | High-dose dexamethasone suppression test required to diagnosis Cushing's syndrome |
| | Cortisol, <5 µg/dL | Cushing's syndrome ruled out |

CAH, congenital adrenal hyperplasia; 17-OHP, 17-hydroxyprogesterone.

**TABLE 68-3.**
**MANAGEMENT OF HIRSUTISM**

| Treatment | Dose | Notes |
|---|---|---|
| Oral contraceptive pills | | Treatment of choice |
|   Progestins | | |
|     Depomedroxy-progesterone acetate | 150 mg IM q3mos | |
|     Medroxyprogesterone | 10–20 mg qd | |
| Spironolactone | 100–200 mg qd | Blocks androgen receptor, suppresses production |
| Glucocorticoids | | Treatment of choice for Cushing's syndrome |
|   Dexamethasone | 0.5 mg qd | |
|   Prednisone | 5–7.5 mg qd | |
| GnRH agonists | | Expensive |
|   Leuprolide (Lupron) | 3.75 mg IM q month | |
| Flutamide | 250 mg qd | Androgen receptor antagonist |
| Finasteride | 5 mg qd | $5\alpha$-reductase inhibitor |
| Ketoconazole | 400 mg qd | Inhibits androgen synthesis |
| | | Elevates liver function tests |
| Cimetidine | 300 mg qid | |
| Eflornithine | Apply bid to facial | Inhibits L-ornithine decarboxylase |
|   Hydrochloride | | FDA approved only for facial hair |
|   (DFMO) [4] | | Side effects: skin stinging |

Note: All dosages are PO unless otherwise noted.

- Immediate hair removal: electrolysis, depilatory creams.
- See Table 68-3.

## SUGGESTED READING

Azziz R. Advances in the evaluation and treatment of unwanted hair growth. *Contemp Obstet Gynecol* 2002;98–106.

Speroff L, Glass RH, Kase NG. *Clinical gynecologic endocrinology and infertility*, 6th edition. Philadelphia: Lippincott Williams & Wilkins, 1999.

Stenchever MA, Droegemueller W, Herbst AL, Mishell DR. *Comprehensive gynecology*. St. Louis: Mosby, 2001.

# 69 Polycystic Ovarian Syndrome

*Polycystic ovarian syndrome is often accompanied by insulin resistance*

## INTRODUCTION

- Hyperandrogenic chronic anovulation
- Onset typically at menarche

## SYMPTOMS

- Menstrual irregularity (amenorrhea, oligomenorrhea)
- Hyperandrogenism (acne, hirsuitism, virilization)
- Obesity
- Enlarged, polycystic ovaries with a thick capsule

## PHYSIOLOGY

See Fig. 69-1.

### Endocrinology

- Increased GnRH secretion with increased LH release.
- LH stimulates theca cells to produce androgens.
- Androgens are converted peripherally to estrone.
- Estrone depresses FSH release, stimulates LH release.
- Ratio of LH to FSH: typically 2–3:1.
- Androgens lead to decreased SHBG.
- Androgenic environment in ovary: follicular atresia, chronic anovulation.
- Condition is cyclic and worsened by obesity.

### Insulin Resistance

- Common in PCOS.
- Leads to hyperinsulinemia and hyperandrogenism.
- Elevated insulin: stimulate insulinlike growth factor-I receptors on thecal cells causing increased androgen production.
- Insulin decreases hepatic synthesis of SHBG.

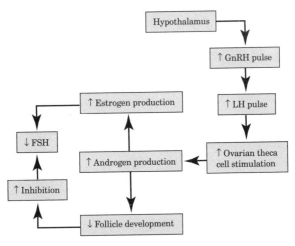

**FIG. 69-1.**
Physiology of polycystic ovarian syndrome.

## CLINICAL MANIFESTATIONS

Evaluation should include a search for

- Menstrual irregularities (oligomenorrhea, amenorrhea)
- Hirsutism (facial hair, alopecia, acne, deepening voice)
- Acanthosis nigricans (velvety discoloration of the skin)
- Infertility
- Ovarian cysts
- Obesity

Patients with polycystic ovarian syndrome are predisposed to HTN and CAD.

## DIAGNOSTIC EVALUATION

- Diagnosis based on symptomatology.
- Ovarian sonography, measurements of FSH and LH not necessary.
- Endometrial biopsy: consider for patients with irregular bleeding.
- Patients with hyperandrogenism should be tested for insulin resistance.
  - 2-hr glucose tolerance test with 75-g glucose load:
    - <140 mg/dL: normal

- 140–199 mg/dL: impaired glucose tolerance
- >200 mg/dL: DM
- Fasting glucose
  - >126 mg/dL: DM

## MANAGEMENT
### Anovulation

- If patient desires pregnancy: ovulation induction
- Dysfunctional uterine bleeding: OCPs

### Hirsutism

- See Chap. 68, Hirsutism

### Obesity

Counsel patient regarding weight loss and diet modification.

### Insulin Resistance

- Metformin and newer insulin sensitizers uncertain.
- Some studies have found increased pregnancy rates in PCOS patients treated with these agents [3,4].

## REFERENCES

1. Speroff L, Glass RH, Kase NG. *Clinical gynecologic endocrinology and infertility.* 6th ed. Philadelphia: Lippincott Williams & Wilkins, 1999.
2. Stenchever MA, Droegemueller W, Herbst AL, Mishell DR. *Comprehensive gynecology.* St. Louis: Mosby, 2001.
3. Dunaif A, Graf M, Mandeli J, et al. Characterization of groups of hyperandrogenic women with acanthosis nigricans, impaired glucose tolerance, and/or hyperinsulinemia. *J Clin Endocrinol Metab* 1987;65:499–507.
4. Nestler JE, Jakubowicz DJ, Evans WS, et al. Effects of metformin on spontaneous and clomiphene-induced ovulation in the polycystic ovary syndrome. *N Engl J Med* 1998;338:1876–1880.

# 70 Hyperprolactinemia

*Hyperprolactinemia causes galactorrhea and amenorrhea*

## PROLACTIN PHYSIOLOGY

- Peptide hormone secreted from anterior pituitary gland.

- Stimulates breast tissue growth and milk production.

- Prolactin secretion tonically inhibited by dopamine produced by hypothalamus.

- Thyrotropin-releasing factor stimulates prolactin secretion.

- Normal level of serum prolactin is 5–27 ng/mL.

## HISTORY

- Galactorrhea, amenorrhea

- CNS compression symptoms: bitemporal hemianopsia, headache

## DIFFERENTIAL DIAGNOSIS

See Table 70-1.

- Physiologic hyperprolactinemia: prolactin elevated secondary to stress, nipple stimulation, exercise, sleep

- Drugs: antipsychotic medications, TCAs, metoclopramide (Reglan), methyldopa (Aldomet, Amodopa), verapamil (Calan, Calan SR, Covera-HS, Isoptin, Isoptin SR, Verelan), cimetidine (Tagamet, Tagamet HB), estrogen

- Prolactinomas: often asymptomatic

- Microadenomas: <1 cm in diameter. Most common pathologic cause of hyperprolactinemia

- Macroadenomas: >1 cm in diameter

- Empty sella syndrome: expansion of subarachnoid space into the sella turcica

- Hypothyroidism: thyrotropin-releasing hormone stimulation of prolactin secretion

## DIAGNOSTIC EVALUATION

See Table 70-2.

## TABLE 70-1.
## DIFFERENTIAL DIAGNOSIS OF HYPERPROLACTINEMIA

Physiologic

 Stress

 Exercise

 Sleep

 Nipple stimulation

 Pregnancy

 Postpartum

 Chest wall disorders (herpes, burns)

Drugs

 Antipsychotics

 TCAs

 Verapamil (Calan, Calan SR, Covera-HS, Isoptin, Isoptin SR, Verelan)

 Methyldopa (Aldomet, Amodopa)

 Reserpine (Serpalan, Serpasil)

 Metoclopramide (Reglan)

 Cimetidine (Tagamet, Tagamet HB)

 Estrogen (HRT, OCPs)

Hypothalamic disease

 Craniopharyngioma

 Dermoid cyst

 TB

 Histiocytosis

 Sarcoidosis

 Pseudotumor cerebri

Anterior pituitary disease

 Prolactinoma

 Other pituitary adenomas

 Metastatic tumors

 Trauma

Other

 Hypothyroidism

 Chronic renal failure

 Ectopic prolactin secretion

 Cirrhosis

### TABLE 70-2.
### DIAGNOSTIC EVALUATION OF HYPERPROLACTINEMIA

History (rule out physiologic causes)

Physical exam (rule out neurologic symptoms)

Prolactin (verify if elevated)

TSH

Creatinine

hCG

CT/MRI (if physiologic causes ruled out)

## Lab

- Prolactin: draw midmorning; repeat elevated level (rule out physiologic elevation)
- TSH: If elevated free $T_4$
- Creatinine
- hCG

### CNS Imaging

- Identify pituitary or hypothalamic lesions
- CT most commonly used; MRI most accurate

### Visual Field Determination

If macroadenoma identified on CNS imaging

## MANAGEMENT

- Treatment indicated if bothersome symptoms, CNS compression, or desire to conceive.
- Patients with a microadenoma and minimal symptoms do not require treatment.

### Dopamine Agonists

- Initial treatment of choice
- Bromocriptine (Parlodel): most commonly used agent
  - Side effects: nausea and vomiting, orthostatic hypotension
  - Initiated before bed; titrate dose
  - Initial dose half of 2.5 mg PO qhs; increase dose q2wks until prolactin level normalizes (usual dose, 2.5 mg bid or tid)

- Cabergoline (Dostinex): alternative medication with long half-life
  - Dosage: 0.25–1.0 mg PO 1–2×/wk
- Medical therapy discontinued 1–2 yrs after normalization of prolactin
- 80–90% relapse; requires reinstituition of therapy

## Transsphenoidal Resection

- Initial response rates are high; late recurrences common
- Transient diabetes insipidous common complication

## Pregnancy

- All patients discontinue treatment
- If CNS symptoms develop: dopamine agonist reinstituted
- 20% of macroadenomas, 1–5% of microadenomas worsen

## FOLLOW-UP
## Prolactin

- Dopamine agonist: obtain at 3, 6, and 12 mos, then yearly
- Expectant management: yearly

## CNS Imaging

- Not repeated unless symptoms of cerebral compression

## SUGGESTED READING

Biller BMK, Luciano A, Crosignani PG, et al. Guidelines for the diagnosis and treatment of hyperprolactinemia. *J Reproduc Med* 1999;44:1075–1084.

Stenchever MA, Droegemueller W, Herbst AL, Mishell DR. *Comprehensive gynecology*. St. Louis: Mosby, 2001.

# 71 Infertility

*Infertility affects 10–15% of couples*

## INTRODUCTION

- Inability to conceive after 1 yr of unprotected intercourse
- Evaluate older couples (age >35) earlier
- Affects 10–15% of reproductive age couples
- Fecundity: probability of achieving pregnancy during one menstrual cycle is 25%

## DIFFERENTIAL DIAGNOSIS

- See Table 71-1.
- Tubal and pelvic factor infertility most commonly result from adhesions, PID, endometriosis.
- Male factor infertility results from any abnormal sperm quantity or function.

## DIAGNOSTIC EVALUATION

- All evaluations include semen analysis, hysterosalpingogram, documentation of ovulation.
- Other optional evaluations are described in Table 71-2.

### Semen Analysis

If abnormality is detected, a repeat analysis is performed in 2 wks–2 mos.

### Ovulation

Document in all women.

### Hysterosalpingogram

- See Table 71-3.
- Determine tubal patency, uterine contour.
- If endometrial cavity normal, hysteroscopy does not need to be performed.
- If fallopian tubes appear abnormal, diagnostic laparoscopy considered.
- May be associated with increased postprocedure fertility rates.

## TABLE 71-1.
## DIFFERENTIAL DIAGNOSIS AND TREATMENT
## OF INFERTILITY

| | | |
|---|---|---|
| Tubal and pelvic factors | 30–40% | Distal tubal obstruction: salpingostomy or fimbrioplasty |
| | | Proximal tubal obstruction: salpingography, tubal canalization |
| | | Severe tubal disease: *in vitro* fertilization |
| | | Mild endometriosis: none |
| | | Moderate to severe endometriosis: surgery |
| Male factors | 30–40% | Intrauterine insemination, intracytoplasmic sperm injection, or sperm aspiration (microsurgical epididymal sperm aspiration or testicular sperm extraction) |
| Anovulation | 10–15% | Ovulation induction |
| Unexplained infertility | 10% | Ovulation induction with IUI |
| Other | 5% | — |

### Postcoital Test

- Evaluate interaction between sperm and cervical mucus (Table 71-4).
- Patients with poor mucus may be given a therapeutic trial of estrogen (CEE, 0.625 mg daily for 8–9 d before ovulation).

### Laparoscopy

- Considered to evaluate abnormal HSG, suspected pelvic adhesions, or endometriosis
- If diagnostic laparoscopy is performed, inject indigo carmine into the uterine cavity and efflux from fallopian tubes evaluated

### Luteal Phase Defect

- When endometrial development lags ≥3 d behind expected pattern
- Diagnosis: timed endometrial biopsy during the luteal phase
- Uncertain if luteal phase defects cause infertility

### MANAGEMENT
### Ovulation Induction

- Performed with a variety of agents (Table 71-5).

## TABLE 71-2.
## SEMEN ANALYSIS AND OVULATION DOCUMENTATION

**Semen analysis**

Abstain from coitus 2–5 d before collection

Collect specimen directly into container

Collect entire specimen

Evaluate motility within 2 hrs of collection

| Parameter | Normal value |
| --- | --- |
| Volume | >2.0 mL |
| pH | 7.2–7.8 |
| Sperm concentration | >20 × $10^6$/mL |
| Total sperm count | >40 × $10^6$/mL |
| Sperm motility | >50% progressive |
| Motility | — |
| Vital staining | >50% live |
| Sperm morphology | >50% normal |
| WBC count | <$10^6$/mL |

**Ovulation documentation**

| | |
| --- | --- |
| Basal body temp | Serum progesterone |
| Document on graph | >10 ng/mL during luteal phase |
| Measure after awakening in a.m. | Home LH kits |
| Temp elevation occurs 2 d after LH surge | Document LH in urine |
| | May replace basal body temp |

## TABLE 71-3.
## HYSTEROSALPINGOGRAM

| | |
| --- | --- |
| Schedule | 2–5 d after menses |
| Prophylactic antibiotics | Consider doxycycline , 200 mg then 100 mg bid × 5 d if a history of PID with dilated tubes |
| Analgesia | NSAID before procedure |
| Contrast agent | |
|     Water soluble | Better visualization of tubal folds, peritoneal irritation, rapidly absorbed |
|     Oil based | Higher pregnancy rate, granuloma formation, embolization |

### TABLE 71-4.
### POSTCOITAL TEST

| | |
|---|---|
| Schedule | Around time of LH surge. Abstain for 2 d before test. |
| Perform | 2–8 hrs after intercourse. |
| Evaluation | |
|    Stretchability (Spinnbarkeit) | Normal, 8–10 cm. |
|    Sperm | Present and motile. |
| | Shaking sperm may indicate sperm antibody, and immunologic testing may be considered. |
|    pH | >7.0. |
|    WBC | Few. |

- Clomiphene (Clomid): estrogen antagonist at the hypothalamus.

- Gonadotropins: human menopausal gonadotropin and FSH stimulate ovulation directly.

- Ovulation occurs in 70–90% with clomiphene, higher with human menopausal gonadotropin.

### TABLE 71-5.
### OVULATION INDUCTION

| Agent | Dosage | Notes |
|---|---|---|
| Clomiphene citrate (Clomid) | Initial: 50 mg qd d 5–9<br><br>Increase by 50 mg each cycle until ovulation<br><br>Max: 250 mg/cycle (some consider 150 mg/d) | Document ovulation with basal body temp or progesterone (>3 ng/mL) 2 wks after last dose<br><br>Multiple gestation 5–10% |
| Human menopausal gonadotropin (FSH and LH, Pergonal; FSH Metrodin) | 1. Baseline U/S<br><br>2. Human menopausal gonadotropin × 3–5 d<br><br>3. Dosing monitored and adjusted by frequent U/S and estradiol levels<br><br>4. 10,000 IU hCG 24 hrs after dominant follicle of sufficient size detected | Use after clomiphene failure or in hypoestrogenic amenorrhea<br><br>Ovarian hyperstimulation 0.1% |
| GnRH | Pulsatile injection by subcutaneous pump | Use for hypothalamic amenorrhea |

**TABLE 71-6.**
**OVARIAN HYPERSTIMULATION SYNDROME**

| Features | Treatment |
|---|---|
| Ascites | Strict input and output |
| Electrolyte disturbances | Electrolyte monitoring and replacement |
| Acute renal failure | Monitor volume status |
| Edema | Monitor respiratory status |
| Ovarian torsion | Is self-limited and will resolve |
| Ovarian rupture | |
| Pleural effusions | |
| Hypovolemia | |
| Hypotension | |
| Weight gain | |
| Hemoconcentration | |
| Pulmonary embolism | |

- Ovarian hyperstimulation syndrome occurs in 1–2% (Table 71-6).

**Intrauterine Insemination**

Intrauterine insemination or intracytoplasmic sperm injection performed for male factor infertility

**Tubal Surgery**

- Distal or fimbrial obstruction: candidates for laparoscopic fimbrioplasty or salpingostomy
- Proximal obstruction: transcervical salpingography may be performed to relieve obstruction

***In Vitro* Fertilization**

- Procedure
- Oocytes aspirated under U/S guidance
- Ova incubated with sperm to allow fertilization
- Fertilized ova cultured
- Embryos then placed into endometrial cavity through a transcervical catheter

- Modifications: gamete intrafallopian transfer, zygote intrafallopian transfer

## SUGGESTED READING

Speroff L, Glass RH, Kase NG. *Clinical gynecologic endocrinology and infertility*, 6th ed. Philadelphia: Lippincott Williams & Wilkins, 1999.

Stenchever MA, Droegemueller W, Herbst AL, Mishell DR. *Comprehensive gynecology*. St. Louis: Mosby, 2001.

# 72       Menopause

Menopause *is defined by amenorrhea for 12 mos*

## INTRODUCTION

- Permanent cessation of menstruation due to loss of ovarian function
- Defined by amenorrhea × 12 mos
- Perimenopause: time preceding menopause to 1 yr after the final menses
- Average age: 51 yrs

## SYMPTOMS

- **Vasomotor instability (hot flashes):** intense heat in the face and thorax often accompanied by visible reddening
- **Genital atrophy**

## OSTEOPOROSIS

- Absolute decrease in amount of bone [1]
- M&M from an increased fracture risk

### Definitions

- Osteoporosis: bone mineral density >2.5 SDs below the mean peak bone mass in young women (T score <–2.5)
- Osteopenia: T score = –1.0 to –2.5

### Pathology

Bone resorption by osteoclasts is greater than bone formation by osteoblasts

### Risk Factors

- Advanced age
- White race
- Family history of osteoporosis
- Personal history of fractures
- Low body weight
- Tobacco use

- Inactivity

- Heavy alcohol use

- Low calcium intake

## Diagnosis

- Dual-energy x-ray absorptiometry: screening test

- Measurements taken at hip and spine and compared to the peak bone mass in young women (T score)

- Other: quantitative U/S, quantitative CT, biochemical markers

## Management

- Initial: increase weight-bearing exercises and calcium supplementation.

- Estrogen therapy is effective in treating and preventing osteoporosis.

- See Table 72-1.

**TABLE 72-1.**
**MANAGEMENT OF OSTEOPOROSIS**

| Treatment | Dosage | Comments |
| --- | --- | --- |
| Calcium | <65 yrs on HRT: 1000 mg/d | |
| | <65 yrs no HRT: 1500 mg/d | |
| | >65 yrs: 1500 mg/d | |
| Estrogen | HRT regimens (see Table 72-2) | 3.5–5.0% increase in bone mineral density at 36 mos [2] |
| Alendronate (Fosamax) | Prevention: 5 mg qd | 47% reduction in fracture risk [3] |
| | Treatment: 10 mg qd, 70 mg once/wk | Side effect: esophagitis |
| | | Take with 6–8 oz water in morning before eating |
| Raloxifene (Evista) | Prevention: 60 mg qd | 30% reduction in vertebral fractures [4] |
| | | Side effects: hot flashes, DVT |
| Calcitonin | 200 IU qd (1 spray) | 36% reduction in vertebral fractures [5] |

DVT, deep venous thrombosis; HRT, hormone replacement therapy.

## HORMONE REPLACEMENT THERAPY (HRT)
### Contraindications
*Cardiovascular Effects*

- Secondary prevention: HRT associated with increase in coronary events in women with underlying CAD and no benefit in prevention [6,7]

- Primary prevention: HRT associated with increase in coronary heart disease in healthy postmenopausal women [8]

*Other Adverse Effects*

- HRT associated with increase in breast cancer (relative risk = 1.26), stroke (relative risk = 1.41) [8]

- Endometrial cancer: patients with intact uterus should receive progesterone + estrogen

- Venous thromboembolism: HRT associated with small increase in risk of thromboembolic disease

**TABLE 72-2.**
**HORMONE REPLACEMENT THERAPY**

| | |
|---|---|
| Unopposed estrogen | |
| Estradiol (Estrace) | 1–2 mg PO qd |
| Conjugated equine estrogens (Premarin) | 0.625–1.25 mg PO qd |
| Estropipate (Ogen, Ortho-Est) | 0.625–5 mg PO qd |
| Estrogen patches | |
| Estradiol (Climara) | 0.05–0.1 mg q wk |
| Estradiol (FemPatch) | 0.025–0.05 mg q wk |
| Estradiol (Estraderm) | 0.05–0.1 mg tiw |
| Estrogen vaginal ring | |
| Estradiol (Estring) | Insert and replace after 90 d |
| Combination estrogen and progestin | |
| Prempro or Premphase (conjugated equine estrogen/medroxyprogesterone) [8] | 0.625 PO mg/2.5–5.0 mg qd |
| FemHRT (ethinyl estradiol/norethindrone acetate) | 5 μg/1 mg qd |
| Activella (estradiol/norethindrone acetate) | 1 mg/0.5 mg |
| Ortho-Prefest (estradiol/norgestimate) | 1 mg/0.09 mg qd |

## Indications

- Based on a large, prospective study [8], many no longer recommend long-term HRT.

- HRT indications: short-term prevention of hot flashes and vaginal atrophy.

## Regimens

- See Table 72-2.

- Intact uterus: estrogen + a progestin to decrease risk of endometrial cancer.

- Estrogen and a progestin may be given continuously or in a cyclic fashion (progestin × 10–14 d/mo).

- Patients receiving cyclic therapy undergo monthly menstruation.

## REFERENCES

1. NIH Consensus Development Panel on Osteoporosis Prevention, Diagnosis, and Therapy. Osteoporosis prevention, diagnosis, and therapy. *JAMA* 2001;285:785–795.
2. The Writing Group for the PEPI Trial. Effects of estrogen or estrogen/progestin regimens on heart disease risk factors in postmenopausal women. *JAMA* 1995;273:199–208.
3. Black DM, Cummings SR, Karpf DB, et al. Randomised trial of effect of alendronate on risk of fracture in women with existing vertebral fractures. *Lancet* 1996;348:1535–1541.
4. Ettinger B, Black D, Mitlak BH, et al. Reduction of vertebral fracture risk in postmenopausal women treated with raloxifene. *JAMA* 1999;282:637–645.
5. Chestnut C, Baylink DJ, Doyle D, et al. Salmon-calcitonin nasal spray prevents vertebral fractures in established osteoporosis. Further interim results of the "PROOF" study. *Osteoporosis Int* 1998;8[Suppl 3]:13.
6. Hulley S, Grady D, Bush T, et al. Randomized trial of estrogen plus progestin for secondary prevention of coronary heart disease in postmenopausal women. *JAMA* 1998;280:605.
7. Herrington DM, Reboussin DM, Brosnihan KB, et al. Effects of estrogen replacement on the progression of coronary-artery atherosclerosis. *N Engl J Med* 2000;343:522–529.
8. Writing Group for the Women's Health Initiative Investigators. Risks and benefits of estrogen plus progestin in healthy postmenopausal women. Principal results from the Women's Health Initiative randomized controlled trial. *JAMA* 2002;288:321–333.

# V

# Gynecologic Oncology

# 73

*Survival tips for gynecologic oncology*

## ROUNDS

- Know your patients.
  - Medical/surgical history
  - Tumor history
  - Medications
- Review staging on all your patients.
- Presentations.
  - Vital signs
  - Input/output
    - Urine output (24 hrs, last shift)
    - Ostomy output
  - Follow up on all labs and studies ordered.
  - Thorough physical exam.
  - Medications.
  - IV fluids.

## WARDS
## Chemotherapy

- Common complications
- Mechanism of action

## Common Problems

- Electrolyte abnormalities
- Bowel obstruction/ileus
- Neutropenia
- Wound infections/breakdown

## Questions

Don't be afraid to ask questions of fellows and senior residents.

## PREOP EVALUATION

- Make sure all labs in order:
  - Type and screen
  - Electrolytes
- Bowel prep
- Preop antibiotics
- Thromboguards or prophylactic heparin

## OR

- Review procedure before surgery.
- Review anatomy.
- Know common complications of procedure.

## STANDARD ADMITTING ORDERS

- Admit: unit/attending
- Diagnosis
  - Primary cancer and stage
  - Secondary diagnosis
- Condition: stable
- Activity: as tolerated/bedrest
- Allergies
- Diet: NPO/regular/ADA 2100
- Vitals: per routine/q hr
- Accurate input and output
- IVF: D5 half NS with 20 mEq KCl transfer 120 cc/hr
- Meds
  - Analgesics [ibuprofen, oxycodone (Percocet), Darvocet (pro-poxyphene), morphine]
  - Stool softener (Colace)
  - Milk of Magnesia/Maalox
  - Antiemetic
  - Consider Pepcid, Benadryl
- Catheters: Foley

# 74 Chemotherapy

*Common antineoplastic agents*

## ANTINEOPLASTIC AGENTS
See Table 74-1.

## ALKYLATING AGENTS
- Cross-link DNA and cause DNA strand breaks
- Acute myelogenous leukemia and myelodysplasia reported 4–10 yrs after treatment
- Dose-limiting side effect: myelosuppression
- Cell-cycle nonspecific

## ANTIMETABOLITES
- Interact with cellular enzymes and modify their activity
- Cell-cycle specific

### Methotrexate (Folex, Rheumatrex, Trexall)
- Inhibits dihydrofolate reductase
- Side effects: interstitial pneumonitis (prednisone), crystalline nephropathy, and renal failure (urine alkalinization)

### 5-Fluorouracil (5-FU)
- Pyrimidine antagonist
- Side effects: stomatitis, diarrhea, chest pain (calcium channel blocker), cerebellar ataxia

## ANTITUMOR ANTIBIOTICS
- Intercalate DNA causing strand breaks, free radicals
- Cell-cycle specific

## PLANT ALKALOIDS
Cell-cycle specific

**TABLE 74-1.**
**ANTINEOPLASTIC AGENTS**

| Agent | Dose Range | Nausea and vomiting | Myelosuppression (days to nadir) | Other toxicity |
|---|---|---|---|---|
| Alkylating agents | | | | |
| Cyclophosphamide (Cytoxan, Neosar) | 60–150 mg/m$^2$ PO qd × 14 d | + | ++ (10–14) | Hemorrhagic cystitis |
| | 500–1500 mg/m$^2$ IV q21d | | | |
| Dacarbazine (DTIC-Dome) | 150–250 mg/m$^2$ IV qd × 5 q21–28 d | +++ | — | Flulike symptoms |
| Hexamethylmelamine (Hexalen) | 260 mg/m$^2$/d PO × 14–21 d | ++ | + (21–28) | Peripheral neuropathy |
| Ifosfamide (Ifex) | 3–5 d q21–28 d | +++ | +++ (7–10) | Hemorrhagic cystitis |
| Melphalan (Alkeran) | 4–8 mg/m$^2$ PO qd × 4 d | — | ++ (10–14) | Neurotoxicity |
| Antimetabolites | | | | |
| 5-Fluorouracil (Efudex, Fluoroplex) | 350–450 mg/m$^2$ IV × 5 d | — | + (7–14) | Phlebitis |
| | 200–1000 mg/m$^2$ infusion × 5 d | | | |
| | 20 mg/m$^2$ qd × 28–56 d with leucovorin | | | |
| Gemcitabine (Gemzar) | 1g/m$^2$ q week × 3 doses q4wks | + | ++ | Peripheral edema |

| Drug | Dose | | | Toxicity |
|---|---|---|---|---|
| Methotrexate (Folex, Rheumatrex, Trexall) | 10–60 mg/m² IV q1–3wks | + | ++ (7–14) | Pneumonitis, Interstitial nephritis |
| Antitumor antibiotics | | | | |
| Bleomycin (Blenoxane) | 10–20 mg/m² SC q wk | — | — | Erythroderma, Pulmonary fibrosis, Allergic reactions |
| Dactinomycin (Actinomycin) | 0.4–1.0 mg/m² IV q wk | ++ | ++ (14–21) | Rash |
| Daunorubicin (DaunoXome) | 45–60 mg/m² IV qd × 3 d | ++ | +++ (7–14) | Vesicant |
| Doxorubicin (Adriamycin, Doxil, Rubex) | 10–60 mg/m² IV q7–28 d | ++ | +++ (7–14) | Cardiotoxic (>500 mg/m²) |
| Mitomycin C (Mutamycin) | 10–20 mg/m² IV q4–6 wks | + | ++ (21–28) | Vesicant |
| Plant alkaloids | | | | |
| Etoposide (VePesid, Etopophos, Toposar) | 50–200 mg/m² PO or IV qd × 5 d | — | ++ (10–14) | — |
| Vinblastine (Velban, Velbe) | 5–10 mg/m² IV q1–4 wks | + | ++ (4–10) | Vesicant |
| Vincristine (Oncovin, Vincasar PFS) | 1–2 mg IV q1–4 wks | — | — | Neuropathy |

*(continued)*

TABLE 74-1.
CONTINUED

| Agent | Dose Range | Nausea and vomiting | Myelosuppression (days to nadir) | Other toxicity |
|---|---|---|---|---|
| Vinorelbine (Navelbine) | 30 mg/m² IV q wk | + | — | — |
| Paclitaxel (Taxol) | 135–250 mg/m² q21d | + | ++ (10–14) | Neuropathy |
| Docetaxel (Taxotere) | 60–100 mg/m² q21d | + | ++ (10–14) | — |
| Platinum compounds | | | | |
| Carboplatin (Paraplatin) | 200–360 mg/m² IV q21–28 d | ++ | ++ (14–28) | — |
| Cisplatin (Platinol, Platinol-AQ) | 20–120 mg/m² IV qd × 1–5 d | +++ | — | Nephropathy |
| | | | | Neuropathy |
| | | | | Ototoxicity |
| Other agents | | | | |
| Hydroxyurea (Droxia, Hydrea) | 500–2000 mg PO qd | — | ++ (7–10) | — |
| Topotecan (Hycamtin) | 1.5 mg/m² IV qd × 5 d q3wks | ++ | +++ (10–14) | Atrophic skin |

Reprinted from Ahya SN, Flood K, Paranjothi S. *The Washington manual of medical therapeutics*, 30th ed. Philadelphia: Lippincott Williams & Wilkins, 2001:440–443.

## Vincristine (Oncovin)

Inhibits microtubule assembly

## Vinblastine (Velban, Velbe)

Inhibits microtubule assembly

## Paclitaxel (Taxol)

- Stabilizes microtubules
- Dissolved in cremophor that may lead to anaphylaxis
- Myelosuppression decreased by shortening infusion time
- Neuropathy decreased by infusing over 24 hrs

## PLATINUM-CONTAINING AGENTS

- Intercalate DNA causing strand breaks
- Cell-cycle specific

## Cisplatin (Platinol, Platinol-AQ)

- Severe nausea and vomiting
- Nephrotoxicity common, preadministration hydration until urine output >100 cc/hr given
- Amifostine (Ethyol) has been used to ameliorate neurotoxicity

## Carboplatin (Paraplatin)

- Less neurotoxicity and nephrotoxicity
- Myelosuppression dose limiting

## OTHER AGENTS
## Topotecan (Hycamtin)

- Inhibits topoisomerase I.
- Myelosuppression is dose limiting.

## Tamoxifen (Nolvadex)

- Selective estrogen receptor modulator.
- Dose 10–20 mg bid.
- Hormonal flare occurs after 7–14 d (bone pain, erythema, hypercalcemia); resolves in 7–10 d.

## SUGGESTED READING

Ahya SN, Flood K, Paranjothi S. *The Washington manual of medical therapeutics*, 30th ed. Philadelphia: Lippincott Williams & Wilkins, 2001.

Young RC, Markman M. Chemotherapy. In: Berek JS, Hacker NF, eds. *Practical gynecologic oncology*, 3rd ed. Philadelphia: Lippincott Williams & Wilkins, 2000:83–115.

# 75 Complications of Chemotherapy

*Chemotherapy can result in life-threatening complications*

## EXTRAVASATION

- Extravasation of chemotherapeutic agents can lead to severe local injury.
- Vesicant chemotherapeutics produce pain, tissue damage, erythema, and discomfort.

### Treatment

- Stop the infusion and aspirate 5 mL blood (remove any residual drug).
- Compresses and neutralization of certain drugs (Table 75-1).
- Observation and analgesia.

## NEUTROPENIA

- Absolute neutrophil count <500/mm³.
- Febrile neutropenic patients are presumed infected.
- Afebrile neutropenic patients should not be treated with empiric antibiotics.

### Diagnostic Evaluation

- Physical exam: indwelling catheters; sinuses; oral, rectal, pelvic, pulmonary, and abdominal exams
- Cultures: blood (peripheral and catheter), urine, sputum, stool
- Lab: CBC, electrolytes, UA, LFTs
- Imaging: CXR, CT (if indicated)

### Treatment

- Initial treatment: empiric antibiotics (Table 75-2) [1]
  - Vancomycin (Vancocin) not used empirically unless oxacillin-resistant *S. aureus* suspected
  - Monotherapy commonly used
- Reverse isolation

**TABLE 75-1.**
## TREATMENT OF EXTRAVASATION OF VESICANTS

| Drug | Compress | Antidote |
| --- | --- | --- |
| Vincristine (Oncovin, Vincasar PFS), vinblastine (Velban, Velbe), and etoposide (VePesid, Etopophos, Toposar) | Hot | Hyaluronidase (150 U/mL) 1–6 mL SC × 1 |
| Doxorubicin (Adriamycin, Doxil, Rubex), daunorubicin (DaunoXome) | Cold | Dimethyl sulfoxide applied topically to vein |
| Dacarbazine (DTIC-Dome) | Hot | Isotonic thiosulfate IV and SC |
| Mitomycin C (Mutamycin), mechlorethamine (Mustargen) | — | Isotonic thiosulfate IV and SC |

- Low-risk patients may be treated as outpatients with a fluoroquinolone or TMP-SMX (Bactrim, Septra)
- G-CSF, 5 µg/kg SC daily after chemotherapy may help prevent neutropenia

### THROMBOCYTOPENIA

- Platelet transfusion considered when platelet count <10,000
- HLA-matched single donor platelets used if available

### ANEMIA

- Symptomatic patients require transfusion.
- Transfusion considered in asymptomatic patients with hemoglobin <7–8 g/dL.
- Erythropoeitin, 150–300 µg/kg SC 3×/wk helps prevent anemia.

### HEMORRHAGIC CYSTITIS

- Complication of cyclophosphamide and ifosfamide
- Toxicity best prevented with prophylactic mesna
- Treatment: continuous bladder irrigation with normal saline. If unresponsive: formalin instillation into bladder

### NAUSEA AND VOMITING
Administer prophylactic antiemetics (Table 75-3)

### STOMATITIS

- Dose-limiting side effect of fluorouracil (Adrucil) and methotrexate (Folex, Rheumatrex, Trexall).

## TABLE 75-2.
## ANTIBIOTIC TREATMENT OF NEUTROPENIA

| | |
|---|---|
| Initial antibiotic | If vancomycin needed |
| | 1. Vancomycin (Vancocin), 1 g IV q12h; and ceftazidime (Fortaz), 1 or 2 g IV q8–12h |
| | Vancomycin not needed |
| | 1. Ceftazidime, 1 or 2 g IV q8–12h or |
| | 2. Cefepime (Maxipime), 0.5–2 g IV q12h or |
| | 3. Imipenem (Primaxin), 250–1000 mg IV q6–8 or |
| | 4. Aminoglycoside + antipseudomonal beta-lactam |
| Afebrile within 3 d | Adjust antibiotic if etiology identified |
| | Low-risk patients: oral quinolone/cefixime (Suprax) |
| | High-risk patients: continue same antibiotics |
| Persistent fever days 4–5 | Reassess/continue antibiotics |
| | No change: continue antibiotics, stop vancomycin |
| | Progressive disease: change antibiotics |
| Persistent fever days 5–7 | Add amphotericin B |
| Duration of treatment | |
| Afebrile by day 3 | Absolute neutrophil count >500/mm$^3$ by day 7: stop after 7 d |
| | Absolute neutrophil count <500/mm$^3$ by day 7 |
| | Low risk: stop when afebrile for 5–7 d |
| | High risk: continue antibiotics |
| Persistent fever | Absolute neutrophil count >500/mm$^3$: stop after 4–5 d |
| | Absolute neutrophil count <500/mm$^3$: continue antibiotics for 2 wks |

Adapted from Hughes WT, Armstron D, Bodey GP, et al. 1997 guidelines for the use of antimicrobial agents in neutropenic patients with unexplained fever. *Clin Infectious Dis* 1997;25:551–573.

- Superimposed *Candida* or HSV infections must be recognized and treated.
- Treatment: see Table 75-4.

## DIARRHEA

Obtain *C. difficile* toxin to rule out pseudomembranous colitis.

## TABLE 75-3.
## ANTIEMETIC THERAPY

Phenothiazines: dopaminergic antagonists

  Prochlorperazine (Compazine), 5–10 mg PO/IV q4–6h, 25 mg PR q3–6h

  Promethazine (Phenergan), 12.5–25 mg PO/IM/PR/IV q4–6h

  Chlorpromazine (Thorazine), 10 mg PO q4–6h

  Trimethobenzamide (Tigan), 100 mg PO/IM q4–6h

Serotonin-receptor (5-HT3) antagonists

  Granisetron (Kytril), 10 µg/kg IV or 1 mg PO q12h × 2 before chemotherapy

  Ondansetron (Zofran), 8–32 mg IV 15–30 mins before or 24 mg PO or 8 mg PO tid

  Dolasetron (Anzemet), 1.8 mg/kg IV or 100 mg PO 30 mins before chemotherapy

Butyrophenones: dopaminergic antagonists

  Droperidol (Inapsine), 1–5 mg IV q4–6h

  Haloperidol (Haldol), 1–3 mg PO or IM q2–4h

Metoclopramide (Reglan), 2–3 mg/kg IV before chemotherapy and q2 × 3 hrs

Scopolamine (Transderm Scop) (transdermal patch), 1 disc (1.5 mg) behind ear q3d

Antihistamines

  Diphenhydramine (Benadryl), 50 mg PO/IV q4–6h

Anxiolytics

  Lorazepam (Ativan), 1–2 mg PO/IV tid–qid

Glucocorticoids

  Dexamethasone (Decadron, Dexamethasone Intensol, Dexone, Hexadrol), 10–30 mg IV before chemotherapy

Adapted from Ahya SN, Flood K, Paranjothi S. *The Washington manual of medical therapeutics*, 30th ed. Philadelphia: Lippincott Williams & Wilkins, 2000.

### Treatment

- Aggressive parenteral hydration
- Antidiarrheal agents: loperamide (Imodium), 4 mg PO, then 2 mg q2h; or diphenoxylate with atropine (Lomotil), 1–2 tabs PO q4h

### ALOPECIA

- Begins 2–4 wks after chemotherapy.

**TABLE 75-4.**
**TREATMENT OF STOMATITIS**

| | |
|---|---|
| Oral rinses | 0.9% NS |
| | Sodium bicarbonate |
| | Chlorhexidine (Peridex, Periogard), 0.12–0.2% |
| Topical anesthetics | Lidocaine (DermaFlex) (viscous, ointment, spray) |
| | Benzocaine (Americaine Topical Anesthetic First Aid Ointment, Americaine Topical Anesthetic Spray) (spray, gel) |
| | Diphenhydramine (Benadryl, Benylin) |
| Combinations | Magnesium aluminum hydroxide/diphenhydramine |
| | Viscous lidocaine ("magic mouthwash") |
| Analgesics | IV/oral opioids |

- Hair regrowth begins 3–6 mos after cessation of chemotherapy.
- Treatment disappointing.

## SUGGESTED READING

Ahya SN, Flood K, Paranjothi S. *The Washington manual of medical therapeutics*, 30th ed. Philadelphia: Lippincott Williams & Wilkins, 2001.

Berman ML, McHale MT. *Cancer treatment*, 5th ed. Philadelphia: WB Saunders, 2001.

## REFERENCE

1. Hughes WT, Armstron D, Bodey GP, et al. 1997 guidelines for the use of antimicrobial agents in neutropenic patients with unexplained fever. *Clin Infect Dis* 1997;25:551–573.

# 76

# Radiation Toxicity

*Radiation-related complications can be debilitating*

## TOXICITY

- Acute toxicity occurs in first 3 mos from mucosal denudation.
- Chronic complications occur >6 mos after treatment from vascular damage.
- Tissue tolerances to radiation are listed in Table 76-1.

## GENITOURINARY COMPLICATIONS

Radiation cystitis, urethral stricture, fistulas

## GI COMPLICATIONS
### Acute Radiation Enteritis

- Nausea and vomiting, crampy abdominal pain, tenesmus, diarrhea, proctitis with rectal pain and bleeding.
- Treatment: rehydration and treatment of diarrhea (Table 76-2).

## TABLE 76-1.
## TISSUE TOLERANCE TO RADIATION

| Tissue | Tolerated dose |
| --- | --- |
| Bladder | 6000–7000 cGy |
| Rectum | 6000-7000 cGy |
| Vaginal mucosa | 7000 cGy |
| Bowel | 6000 cGy |
| Cervix | >12,000 cGy |
| Kidney | 2000–2300 cGy |
| Liver | 2500–3500 cGy |

Reprinted from Stenchever MA, Droegemueller W, Herbst AL, Mishell DR. *Comprehensive gynecology*, 4th ed. St. Louis: Mosby, 2001:832, with permission.

## TABLE 76-2.
## TREATMENT OF RADIATION ENTERITIS

Diphenoxylate/atropine (Lomotil), 1–2 tabs q4h

Loperamide (Imodium), 4 mg PO q4h and 2 mg with each stool

Kaopectate, 30–60 cc PO with bowel movements

Paregoric, 1 tsp PO qid

Donnatal, 1–2 tabs q4h

Cholestyramine, 1 package PO with meals

- Steroid enemas may relieve proctitis.
- Symptoms usually resolve after 2–3 wks.

### Chronic Radiation Enteritis

- Develops in 5–15% of patients
- Similar to acute enteritis + obstruction, fistulas, bowel perforation
- Treatment: symptomatic as described for acute enteritis; surgery may be required

### SUGGESTED READING

Berek JS, Hacker NF. *Practical gynecologic oncology*, 3rd ed. Philadelphia: Lippincott Williams & Wilkins, 2000.

Stenchever MA, Droegemueller W, Herbst AL, Mishell DR. *Comprehensive gynecology*, 4th ed. St. Louis: Mosby, 2001.

# 77

# Epithelial Ovarian Cancer

*Epithelial neoplasms are the most common ovarian carcinomas*

## INTRODUCTION

- 23,300 new cases, 13,900 deaths from ovarian cancer in 2002

- Classification: epithelial neoplasms (85%), germ cell tumors (10%), sex cord-stromal tumors (5%)

- Mean age at diagnosis: 61

*BHcG ⊥ AFP Also*
*NARkotis of*
*use*
*LDH*

## EPIDEMIOLOGY
### Risk Factors

- Low parity, infertility, early menarche, late menopause, anovulatory disorders

- Family history of breast or colon cancer

- OCPs protective (relative risk, 0.5 after 5 yrs)

### Genetic Risk

- 5–10% hereditary

- BRCA 1 and BRCA 2 mutations

  - Increased risk breast, ovarian cancer

  - Younger, family history, Ashkenazi Jewish descent

### Management of High-Risk Patients

- Genetic counseling, possible genetic testing

- Offer OCPs

- TVS (q6–12mos)

- Periodic mammography, colonoscopy, and endometrial sampling

- Consider prophylactic oopherectomy (if documented BRCA mutation)

## SCREENING

- General population screening: not recommended

- Ca 125: antigen present on coelomic epithelium

  - Elevated in 50% of stage I disease, 90% advanced disease

  - Low specificity, often elevated in benign diseases

**308**

## PATHOLOGY

- Surface epithelial tumors may be benign, malignant, or borderline.

- Borderline ovarian tumors (tumors of low malignant potential [LMP]): represent 15% of ovarian tumors, occur in younger women, improved survival.

- Serous tumors: 40–50% of malignant epithelial tumors, often bilateral.

- Endometrioid tumors: 15–25% of malignant epithelial tumors, borderline tumors rare.

- Mucinous tumors: 6–16% of malignant epithelial tumors.

  - Pseudomyxoma peritonei: mucin fills abdominopelvic cavity.

- Clear cell tumors: 5–11% of epithelial cancers, aggressive.

- Transitional cell (Brenner) tumors: composed of transitional epithelium.

- Mixed carcinomas: two or more histologies.

## HISTORY

- GI complaints (nausea and vomiting, early satiety, bloating)

- Increased abdominal girth

## PHYSICAL EXAM

- Pelvic exam (adnexal mass)

- Abdominal exam (ascites)

- Pulmonary exam (pleural effusion)

## DIAGNOSTIC EVALUATION

Diagnosis usually made during surgical exploration

### Pelvic Mass

- Management based on the patient's age and the mass size

- Premenarchal/postmenopausal: surgical exploration

- Reproductive age with >8-cm mass: surgical exploration

- Reproductive age with <8-cm mass: observation

- All patients require TVS initially and at follow-up

### Paracentesis

- Consider in patients with ascites.

- Negative cytology does not rule out ovarian carcinoma.

## TABLE 77-1.
## STAGING AND SURVIVAL OF EPITHELIAL OVARIAN CANCER

| Stage | Location | 5-yr survival (%) |
|-------|----------|-------------------|
| I | Confined to ovary | 93 |
| IA | Limited to one ovary; no ascites, capsule intact | |
| IB | Limited to both ovaries; no ascites, capsule intact | |
| IC | IA or IB with ascites or capsule ruptured | |
| II | Pelvic extension | 70 |
| IIA | Metastasis to uterus or tubes | |
| IIB | Extension to other pelvic tissues | |
| IIC | IIA or IIB with ascites or capsule ruptured | |
| III | Peritoneal implants outside pelvis, positive retroperitoneal | 37 |
| | Lymph nodes, omental, small bowel or superficial liver metastasis | |
| IIIA | Microscopic abdominal disease, nodes negative | |
| IIIB | Abdominal implants <2 cm, nodes negative | |
| IIIC | Abdominal implants >2 cm or positive nodes | |
| IV | Distant metastasis, cytologically positive pleural effusion, parenchymal liver metastasis | 25 |

## Preop Evaluation

- Lab: CA 125, CBC, electrolytes
- Imaging: optional CXR, CT, MRI, IV pyelogram
- Colorectal evaluation: colonoscopy or barium enema
- Staging: surgical (Table 77-1)

## MANAGEMENT

- Initial treatment of all stages: staging laporotomy with cytoreductive surgery.
- See Table 77-2.
  - Staging laparotomy: multiple biopsies from peritoneum, diaphragm
  - Cytoreductive surgery: resection of as much tumor as is feasible

## TABLE 77-2.
## MANAGEMENT OF EPITHELIAL OVARIAN CANCER

Early-stage disease

| | |
|---|---|
| Low risk (stage IA, IB) | Staging/TAH/BSO |
| High risk (stage IA, IB grade 2 and 3, stage IC) | Staging/TAH/BSO |
| | Adjuvant: platinum/paclitaxel chemotherapy |

Advanced-stage disease (II–IV)    Staging/TAH/BSO/cytoreduction

                                        Adjuvant: platinum/paclitaxel chemotherapy

                                        Alternate: whole abdominal radiation (optimal reduction)

Borderline tumors

| | |
|---|---|
| Early stage (stage I) | Staging/TAH/BSO or unilateral oopherectomy |
| Advanced stage (II–IV) | Staging/TAH/BSO/cytoreduction |

BSO, bilateral salpingo-oopherectomy; TAH, total abdominal hysterectomy.

- Optimal cytoreduction (visible tumor <1 cm) associated with improved survival [1]
- Stage IC–IV: require adjuvant therapy.
- Adjuvant therapy.
  - Chemotherapy: platinum compound and paclitaxel first line [2]
  - Radiation: feasible if limited gross residual disease
- Borderline tumors.
  - Staging laparotomy with cytoreductive surgery
  - Extensive sampling mandatory to rule out invasive neoplasm
  - Unilateral oopherectomy or cystectomy adequate if confined to ovary
  - 5-yr survival: 80–90%
  - Adjuvant treatment not needed

## RECURRENT DISEASE

- Second-look surgery: performed after frontline surgery and adjuvant therapy to assess disease status. Results are prognostic, but no survival benefit.

- Secondary cytoreduction: consider in highly selected patients with long disease-free interval (>2 yrs) with isolated recurrence.

- Chemotherapy: platinum-sensitive tumors (>12 mo interval between initial treatment and relapse) retreated with platinum-containing compound.

## COMPLICATIONS
### Bowel Obstruction

Usually secondary to mechanical blockage from peritoneal disease

### *History and Physical Exam*

- Abdominal pain (crampy)

- Nausea and vomiting

- Abdominal distention

- Hyperactive bowel sounds

- Decreased flatus

### *Differential Diagnosis*

- Ileus: similar symptoms, abdominal pain often continuous with bowel sounds absent or decreased.

- Bowel ischemia must be ruled out.

- Peritonitis present with tachycardia, fever and rigidity.

### *Diagnosis*

- Abdominal films: dilated loops of bowel with air fluid levels. Free air under the diaphragm is a sign of perforation.

- Barium enema: define location of large bowel obstruction.

- Lab: CBC, electrolytes.

### *Treatment*

- IV hydration, electrolye replacement

- Decompression: NG tube

- Parenteral antiemetics

- Surgical emergencies: bowel ischemia, perforation, dilation to >12 cm

- Surgical bypass/resection considered in context of life expectancy

### Ascites

Therapeutic, large volume paracentesis undertaken for patient comfort

## Pleural Effusion

Thoracentesis or chest tube placement with pleurodesis for recurrent effusions

## FOLLOW-UP

* Evaluated q3mos × 2 yrs, then q6mos × 3 yrs.

* CA 125 can be used to predict progression or recurrence. Negative CA 125 does not rule out recurrence.

* CT scanning valuable adjunct (45% false-negative rate).

## REFERENCES

1. Hoskins WJ, McGuire WP, Brady MF, et al. The effect of diameter of largest residual disease on survival after primary cytoreductive surgery in patients with suboptimal residual epithelial ovarian carcinoma. *Am J Obstet Gynecol* 1994;170:974–979.
2. McGuire WP, Hoskins WJ, Brady MF, et al. Cyclophosphamide and cisplatin compared with paclitaxel and cisplatin in patients with stage III and stage IV ovarian cancer. *N Engl J Med* 1996;334:1–6.

# 78

# Nonepithelial Ovarian Cancer

*Nonepithelial ovarian tumors often secrete a tumor marker*

## GERM CELL TUMORS
### Introduction

- 10% of ovarian cancers
- Derived from primordial germ cells
- Affect young women

### HISTORY

- Rapidly enlarging abdominopelvic mass
- Acute abdominal pain (secondary to torsion, rupture, hemorrhage)
- Menstrual irregularities

### PHYSICAL EXAM

Pelvic exam: adnexal mass

### DIAGNOSTIC EVALUATION

- Diagnosis requires exploratory laparotomy
- Lab: hCG, AFP, LDH, CBC
- Imaging: CXR, optional abdominal and pelvic CT
- Karyotype (rule out dysgenetic gonad)

### STAGING

Similar to epithelial ovarian cancer

### PATHOLOGY
#### Dysgerminoma

- Most common malignant germ cell tumor
- Tumor marker: LDH
- 5% arise from dysgenetic gonads

#### Mature Teratoma (Dermoid Cyst)

- Most common of all ovarian neoplasms
- Contain tissue from all three germ layers

- Struma ovarii: variant where functional thyroid tissue present
- Malignant element arises in 2%

## Immature Teratoma

Graded based on amount and differentiation of neuroepithelial elements

## Endodermal Sinus Tumors (Yolk Sac Tumors)

- Schiller-Duval bodies: small glomeruluslike structures
- Tumor marker: AFP

## Embryonal Carcinoma

- Tumor markers: hCG, AFP
- Choriocarcinoma
- Tumor marker: hCG

## Mixed Germ Cell Tumors

## MANAGEMENT

- Treatment begins with surgical staging.
- Conservative fertility-sparing surgery for patients who desire future childbearing.
- Initial and adjuvant treatment is shown in Table 78-1.

## OUTCOME

5-yr survival: dysgerminomas (90–100%), immature teratomas (70–80%), endodermal sinus tumors (60–70%)

## SEX CORD–STROMAL TUMORS
### Introduction

- 5% ovarian malignancies
- Derived from ovarian sex cords and stromal tissue

## GRANULOSA CELL TUMOR

- Mean age at diagnosis: 52
- Call-Exner bodies: rosettes with cells with coffee-bean groove in nucleus
- Tumor marker: inhibin
- Estrogen secreted: sexual pseudoprecocity, endometrial hyperplasia and carcinoma

**TABLE 78-1.**
**MANAGEMENT OF NONEPITHELIAL OVARIAN CANCER**

| | |
|---|---|
| Germ cell tumors | |
| Dysgerminoma | |
| Early stage (IA and IB) | Staging/USO |
| Advanced stage (IC–IV) | Staging/USO/cytoreduction |
| | Adjuvant: bleomycin/etoposide/ cisplatin [1] |
| Other germ cell tumors | |
| Immature teratoma (stage IA, grade 1) | Staging/USO |
| All others | Staging/USO/cytoreduction |
| | Adjuvant: bleomycin/etoposide/ cisplatin |
| Sex cord–stromal tumors | |
| Granulosa cell tumor | Staging/cytoreduction/endome-trial sampling |
| Sertoli-Leydig cell tumor | Staging/cytoreduction |

USO, unilateral salpingo-oopherectomy.

- Treatment: staging laparotomy, cytoreductive surgery, endometrial evaluation
- Prolonged survival with late recurrences common

### SERTOLI-LEYDIG TUMORS

- Arise from testicular-type tissue.
- Androgens secreted: virilization (70–85%).
- Treatment: staging, unilateral salpingo-oopherectomy if localized disease present. Adjuvant therapy uncertain.

### SUGGESTED READING

Williams SD. Ovarian germ cell tumors: an update. *Sem Oncol* 1998;25:407–413.

### REFERENCE

1. Williams SD, Birch R, Einhorn LH. Treatment of disseminated germ cell tumors with cisplatin, bleomycin and either vinblastine or etoposide. *N Engl J Med* 1987;316:1435–1440.

# 79

# Cervical Intraepithelial Neoplasia

*Cervical intraepithelial neoplasia (CIN) can be a precursor of cervical cancer*

## INTRODUCTION

CIN: premalignant change of cervical epithelial cells diagnosed by cervical cytology (Pap smear)

## RISK FACTORS

- HPV infection
- Young age at first intercourse, multiple sex partners
- Tobacco use
- High parity
- Low socioeconomic status
- Early childbearing
- Immunosuppression
- High-risk male partners

## SCREENING

- Screening: Pap smear
- Begin: 18 yrs or time of first intercourse
- Interval: annual (q3yrs if low risk with 2 negative smears)
- Cessation [1]
  - 65 if normal smears (U.S. Preventive Services task force)
  - Indefinite (ACOG, ACS)
- After hysterectomy
  - May consider cessation
  - Vaginal cuff smears q5yrs (ACOG)
- Liquid-based cytology
  - Increases detection and decreases atypical squamous cell of undetermined significance

**TABLE 79-1.**
**CLASSIFICATION AND MANAGEMENT OF**
**ABNORMAL CYTOLOGY**

| Classification | Recommended management | Chance of cervical intraepithelial neoplasia 2 or 3 on biopsy (%) | Special populations |
|---|---|---|---|
| Atypical squamous cells of undetermined significance | HPV testing<br><br>Repeat cytology<br><br>Immediate colposcopy | 5–17 | Postmenopausal: vaginal estrogen and repeat cytology |
| Atypical squamous cells of undetermined significance, cannot exclude high-grade squamous intraepithelial lesion | Immediate colposcopy | 24–94 | — |
| Low-grade squamous intraepithelial lesion | Immediate colposcopy | 15–30 | Postmenopausal: repeat cytology (6–12 mos) or HPV testing (12 mos)<br><br>Adolescents: repeat cytology (6–12 mos) or HPV testing (12 mos) |
| High-grade squamous intraepithelial lesion | Immediate colposcopy with endocervical curettage | 70–75 | Pregnant: avoid endocervical curettage |

- Increased cost
- HPV testing

## CLASSIFICATION

- Based on Bethesda system (Table 79-1).
- Classification based on Pap smear determines further management.
- "Reflex" HPV testing may be performed on liquid-based cytology samples.
- Diagnosis (Fig. 79-1).

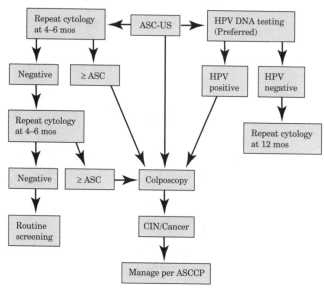

**FIG. 79-1.**
Management of atypical squamous cells of undetermined significance.

## DIAGNOSIS
### Colposcopy

- Transformation zone visualized after applying 3% acetic acid

- Identify: acetowhite epithelium, abnormal vessels (punctation or mosaic pattern)

- Endocervical curettage, directed biopsies performed

### Cone Biopsy

- Further evaluate abnormal cervical cytology

- Performed by loop electroexcision procedure, laser, or surgical (cold knife conization)

## TREATMENT MODALITIES

- Consider for cervical intraepithelial neoplasia 1–3 on biopsy.

- Ablation: cryotherapy, laser.

- Excision: loop electroexcision procedure, cold knife conization.

- See Figs. 79-2 and 79-3.

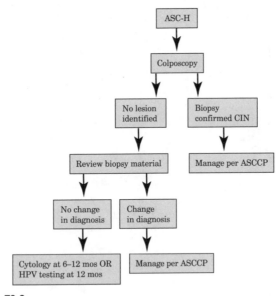

**FIG. 79-2.**
Management of atypical squamous cells of undetermined significance, cannot exclude high-grade squamous intraepithelial lesion.

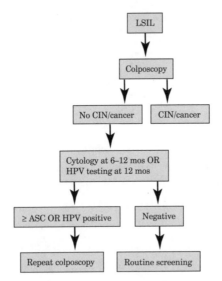

**FIG. 79-3.**
Management of high-grade squamous intraepithelial lesion.

## SUGGESTED READING

Wright TC, Cox JT, Massad LS, et al. 2001 consensus guidelines for the management of women with cervical cytological abnormalities. *JAMA* 2002;287:2120–2129.

Solomon D, Schiffman M, Tarone R, et al. Comparison of three management strategies for patients with atypical squamous cells of undetermined significance: baseline results from a randomized trial. *J Natl Cancer Inst* 2001;93:293–299.

## REFERENCE

1. Sawaya GF, Adalsteinn DB, Washington AE, et al. Current approaches to cervical-cancer screening. *N Engl J Med* 2001;344:1603–1607.

# 80

# Cervical Cancer

*Cervical cancer is the second most common cancer worldwide*

## INTRODUCTION

- 13,000 new cases; 4100 deaths in 2002
- Mean age at diagnosis: 51.4

## RISK FACTORS

- HPV: found in most cervical neoplasms
- High-risk genotypes: HPV 16, 18, 31, 45
- Cervical intraepithelial neoplasia
- Other: smoking (active and passive), multiple sex partners, early age at first intercourse, immunosuppression, low socioeconomic status

## PATHOLOGY

- Squamous cell carcinoma: 90% of invasive cervical carcinomas
- Adenocarcinoma: often arise in endocervical canal
- Adenocarcinoma *in situ*: often associated with adenocarcinoma, cervical intraepithelial neoplasia
- Adenosquamous carcinoma: prognosis may be worse than squamous carcinomas
- Glassy cell carcinoma: poorly differentiated adenocarcinoma
- Villoglandular adenocarcinoma: occurs in young women; good prognosis
- Small cell carcinoma: aggressive, early metastasis

## HISTORY

- Often found on cytology in asymptomatic women
- Irregular vaginal bleeding (often postcoital)
- Vaginal discharge
- Pelvic pain

## PHYSICAL EXAM

- Speculum, bimanual, and rectovaginal exams to assess tumor size and parametrial involvement

- Supraclavicular/inguinal lymph node palpation

## DIAGNOSTIC EVALUATION

- Gross lesion: cervical biopsy

- No gross lesion: colposcopy, endocervical curettage, directed biopsy

- Microinvasive disease: cone biopsy

- Imaging: optional CT, MRI, PET, IV pyelogram, lymphangiography, cystoscopy, proctoscopy

## SPREAD

- Most commonly spreads by direct extension

- Lymphatic spread: parametrial, obturator, iliac, paraaortic nodes

## STAGING

- Clinical staging (Table 80-1)

- Acceptable staging procedures: colposcopy, endocervical curettage, hysteroscopy, cystoscopy, proctoscopy, IV pyelogram, x-ray

## MANAGEMENT

See Table 80-2.

- Radical hysterectomy complications: UTI, DVT, pulmonary embolism, fistulas, lymphocyst, ileus, prolonged bladder dysfunction, lymphedema, sexual dysfunction

### Recurrent Disease

- Local recurrences: radiation

- Central pelvic recurrences (after prior radiation): pelvic exenteration

- Distant metastasis: chemotherapy

### Cervical Cancer in Pregnancy

- Stage for stage survival is identical to nonpregnant patients.

- Abnormal Pap smear: evaluated with colposcopy and directed biopsy without ECC.

- Microinvasive disease.
  - Evaluate with cone biopsy

TABLE 80-1.
## STAGING AND SURVIVAL OF CERVICAL CANCER

| Stage | | | 5-yr survival (%) |
|---|---|---|---|
| I | | Confined to cervix | |
| | IA | Microscopic lesions (no visible tumor) | |
| | | IA1 Stromal invasion < 3 mm and extension <7 mm | 95 |
| | | IA2 Stromal invasion 3–5 mm and extension <7 mm | 95 |
| | IB | Clinically visible or microscopic greater than IA | 80 |
| | | IB1 visible lesion <4 cm | |
| | | IB2 visible lesion >4 cm | |
| II | | Invades beyond uterus, not to pelvic wall or lower one-third of vagina | |
| | IIA | No obvious parametrial involvement, upper two-thirds of vagina | 66 |
| | IIB | Obvious parametrial involvement | 64 |
| III | | Extends to pelvic wall, lower one-third of vagina or hydronephrosis | |
| | IIIA | Lower one-third of vagina, no extension to pelvic wall | 33 |
| | IIIB | Extension to pelvic wall or hydronephrosis | 39 |
| IV | | Beyond pelvis or to mucosa of bladder or rectum | |
| | IVA | Spread to adjacent organs | 17 |
| | IVB | Spread to distant organs | 9 |

- Stage IA1 disease: treat postpartum
- Stage IA2 disease: treat as described below
- Microinvasive disease diagnosed in third trimester: evaluate post-partum
- Gestational age <24 wks.
  - Primary surgery (stage IA2–IIA) or radiotherapy (IIB–IVB) at time of diagnosis
  - Usually undergo spontaneous abortion, otherwise hysterotomy
- Gestational age >24 wks.
  - May elect treatment after delivery

**TABLE 80-2.**
**MANAGEMENT OF CERVICAL CANCER**

| | |
|---|---|
| Microinvasive disease | |
| Stage IA1 | 1. Cone biopsy (if positive margins or endocervical curettage, repeat cone or modified radical hysterectomy/lymph node dissection) |
| | 2. Extrafascial hysterectomy |
| | 3. Intracavitary radiation (medically unfit) |
| Stage IA2 | 1. Modified radical hysterectomy/lymph node dissection |
| | 2. Intracavitary radiation (medically unfit) |
| Early-stage disease | |
| Stage IB1/IIA | 1. Radical hysterectomy/LND |
| | Adjuvant: radiation + cisplatin ± 5-fluorouracil (if positive lymph node, margins or parametrium) |
| | 2. Radiation |
| Stage IB 2 | Radiation + cisplatin ± 5-fluorouracil |
| Advanced stage disease | |
| Stage IIB–IVA | Radiation (external/brachytherapy) + cisplatin ± 5-fluorouracil |
| Stage IVB | Palliative radiation |

- Antenatal corticosteroids administered and classic cesarean performed at time of fetal lung maturity

## COMPLICATIONS
### Cervical Bleeding
- Initial: vaginal pack soaked with ferric subsulfate (Monsel's solution).
  - Remove if febrile
  - Other: ring implant, uterine artery embolization
- Bleeding often controlled once external beam therapy begun.

### Obstructive Uropathy
- Secondary to tumor obstruction or radiation fibrosis.
- Kidney function evaluated by renal scan.
- Initial treatment: cystoscopy with retrograde ureteral stent placement.

- If stenting unsuccessful: percutaneous nephrostomy.

- If no residual renal function demonstrated on renal scan-consider hemodialysis.

### Radiation Complications

### OUTCOME
### Follow-Up

- q3mos × 2 yrs, q6mos × 3 yrs, then annually

- Pap smear performed at every visit

### SUGGESTED READING

National Institutes of Health. Consensus statement 102. *Cervical cancer*. April, 1996.

Morris M, Eifel PJ, Lu J, et al. Pelvic radiation with concurrent chemotherapy compared with pelvic and paraaortic radiation for high-risk cervical cancer. *N Engl J Med* 1999;340:1137–1143.

Rose PG, Bundy B, Watkins EB, et al. Concurrent cisplatin-based radiotherapy and chemotherapy for locally advanced cervical cancer. *N Engl J Med* 1999;340:1144–1153.

American College of Obstetricians and Gynecologists. *Diagnosis and treatment of cervical carcinomas. ACOG Practice Bulletin 35*. Washington, DC: ACOG, 20042.

# 81 Endometrial Hyperplasia

*Endometrial hyperplasia is a precursor of endometrial cancer*

## INTRODUCTION

- Usually results from unopposed estrogenic stimulation of endometrium
- Untreated, may progress to endometrial cancer
- Risk factors: anovulatory disorders, unopposed estrogen, tamoxifen, obesity

## HISTORY

- Vaginal bleeding
- Many asymptomatic

## DIAGNOSTIC EVALUATION

- **Endometrial biopsy:** highly accurate
- **U/S:** assess endometrial thickness
- Endometrial thickness of <5 mm has high negative predictive value
- **Dilation and curettage:** gold standard for diagnosis
- Combined with hysteroscopy to improve detection of benign lesions

## PATHOLOGY

- **Simple hyperplasia:** dilated glands without cytological atypia; progression to cancer: 1–5%
- **Complex hyperplasia:** crowded glands and little stroma; progression to cancer: 3–15%
- **Atypical hyperplasia:** hyperplasia with cellular atypia; progression to cancer: 8–30% [1]

## MANAGEMENT

See Fig. 81-1.

### Medical Management

- Progestin: treatment of choice. Initial treatment: medroxyprogesterone (Provera), 10–20 mg qd × 11–14 d/mo.

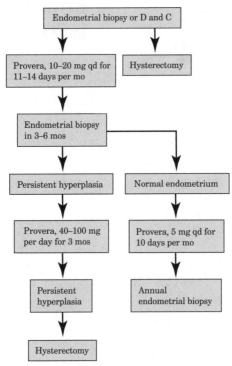

**FIG. 81-1.**
Management of endometrial hyperplasia. (Adapted from Berek JS, Hacker NF. *Practical gynecologic oncology*, 3rd ed. Philadelphia: Lippincott Williams & Wilkins, 2000:422.)

- Perform dilation and curettage before treatment if atypical hyperplasia diagnosed on biopsy.

- Endometrial biopsy repeated in 3–6 mos.

- If hyperplasia does not resolve: high-dose progestin therapy: Provera, 40–100 mg qd × 11–14 d/mo

- Patients desiring pregnancy: ovulation induction (clomiphene citrate [Clomid])

## Surgical Management

- Hysterectomy

- Appropriate if childbearing completed, failed medical management

## SUGGESTED READING

Berek JS, Hacker NF. *Practical gynecologic oncology*, 3rd ed. Philadelphia: Lippincott Williams & Wilkins, 2000.

## REFERENCE

1. Kurman RJ, Kaminski PF, Norris HJ. Behavior of endometrial hyperplasia: a long-term study of "untreated" hyperplasias in 170 patients. *Cancer* 1985;56:403.

# 82 Uterine Cancer

*Endometrial cancer is the most common gynecologic cancer in the United States*

## INTRODUCTION

- 39,300 new cases; 6600 deaths in 2002
- 95% endometrial cancers, 3–5% are uterine sarcomas
- Mean age at diagnosis: 61

## ENDOMETRIAL CANCER
### Risk Factors

- **Unopposed estrogen:** early menarche, late menopause, obesity, anovulatory disorders.
- **Endometrial hyperplasia.**
- **Tamoxifen:** increases endometrial cancer, hyperplasia, polyps.
- Routine endometrial sampling not indicated.
- **Hereditary nonpolyposis colorectal cancer syndrome:** 20–43% lifetime risk of endometrial cancer. Yearly endometrial sampling may be warranted.

### Pathology

- **Endometrioid adenocarcinoma:** 75% of endometrial cancers
  - Grading: 1 (<5% solid), 2 (6–50% solid), 3 (>50% solid)
- **Uterine papillary serous carcinoma:** 5–10% of carcinomas
  - Aggressive: deep invasion, early peritoneal spread
  - All classified as high-grade lesions
- **Clear cell carcinoma:** <5% of endometrial carcinomas
  - High grade, poor prognosis
- **Mucinous carcinoma**
- **Mixed carcinoma**
- **Undifferentiated carcinoma**

### History

- Postmenopausal bleeding (90%)

- Pyometra or hematometra if cervical stenosis present

## Physical Exam

Pelvic and rectovaginal exams (often unremarkable)

## Diagnostic Evaluation

### Endometrial Sampling

- First step in evaluating abnormal vaginal bleeding
- Sensitivity: >90%
- If sample negative and suspicion for endometrial cancer remains: fractional curettage

### Pap Smear

Normal or abnormal endometrial cells on Pap smear require further evaluation.

### Fractional Dilation and Curettage

- Gold standard for diagnosis
- Hysteroscopy useful for evaluating polyps, benign uterine processes

### Transvaginal Ultrasound

- Assess endometrial thickness
- Cutoff 5 mm: sensitivity >95% for detecting endometrial hyperplasia and cancer
- Sonohysterography: detection of polyps, leiomyomas

### Postmenopausal Vaginal Bleeding

- Evaluation: pelvic exam, Pap smear, endometrial sampling, endocervical curettage
- Exogenous estrogens and atrophic endometritis most common

### Spread

- Direct extension into the myometrium then serosa into peritoneal cavity
- Lymphatic spread: pelvic and paraaortic nodes

### Staging

Surgical (Table 82-1)

## Management

### General Principles

- All medically fit patients initially treated surgically.
- Adjuvant therapy recommended based on surgical findings.

**TABLE 82-1.**
**STAGING AND SURVIVAL OF ENDOMETRIAL CANCER**

| Stage | | 5-yr survival (%) |
|---|---|---|
| I | | |
| IA | Tumor limited to endometrium | 91 |
| IB | Invasion to less than one-half of myometrium | 88 |
| IC | Invasion to more than one-half of myometrium | 81 |
| II | | |
| IIA | Endocervical glandular involvement | 77 |
| IIB | Cervical stromal invasion | 67 |
| III | | |
| IIIA | Invades seros and adnexa or positive peritoneal cytology | 60 |
| IIIB | Vaginal metastasis | 41 |
| IIIC | Pelvic/paraaortic lymph node metastasis | 32 |
| IV | | |
| IVA | Invasion of bladder or bowel mucosa | 20 |
| IVB | Distant metastasis, abdominal spread, inguinal lymph nodes | 5 |

- Radiotherapy if surgery contraindicated for medical reasons.
- Pelvic and paraaortic lymphadenectomy: performed if >50% myometrial invasion (stage IC or higher), cervical extension, grade 3 lesions, tumors >2 cm in size and clear cell or papillary serous tumors (some perform on all patients).
- See Table 82-2.

*Recurrent Disease*

- Hormonal therapy: progestational agents
- Chemotherapy: doxorubicin, cisplatin

**Prognosis**
*Follow-Up*

- q3mos × 2 yrs, q6mos × 3 yrs, then yearly
- Obtain Pap smear at each visit, chest x-ray annually

## TABLE 82-2.
## MANAGEMENT OF ENDOMETRIAL CANCER

Early stage disease

| | |
|---|---|
| Stage IA, IB (grade 1, 2) | TAH/BSO ± LND |
| | Adjuvant: none |
| Stage IA, IB (grade 3), IC | TAH/BSO/LND |
| | Adjuvant: whole pelvis or vaginal vault radiation or none |
| Stage II | 1. Radical or modified radical hysterectomy/LND |
| | Adjuvant: whole pelvis or vaginal vault radiation or none |
| | 2. Whole pelvis radiation with brachytherapy |
| | Adjuvant: TAH/BSO (in 4–6 wks) |

Advanced stage disease

| | |
|---|---|
| Stage IIIA, IIIC | TAH/BSO/LND/omentectomy |
| | Adjuvant: whole pelvis or whole abdomen radiation |
| Stage IIIB | 1. TAH/BSO/LND/omentectomy |
| | Adjuvant: whole pelvis radiation |
| | 2. Whole pelvis radiation with brachytherapy |
| | Adjuvant: TAH/BSO (in 4–6 wks) |
| Stage IV | Individualized (radiation, hormonal agents, surgery) |

BSO, bilateral salpingo-oophorectomy; LND, lymph node dissection; TAH, total abdominal hysterectomy.

### *Hormone Replacement Therapy*

- No evidence that HRT either increases recurrences or decreases survival

## UTERINE SARCOMAS
### Introduction

- Only known risk factor: exposure to pelvic radiation
- Staging similar to endometrial carcinoma

### Pathology

Aggressive with direct extension and early hematogenous metastasis

## *Leiomyosarcoma*

- 30% of uterine sarcomas
- Most common in women aged 45–55
- Usually arise from uterine smooth muscle, not preexisting leiomyoma
- Presentation: rapidly enlarging uterine mass, endometrial growth is unusual
- Diagnosis often not made preoperatively

## *Endometrial Stromal Sarcomas*

- 15% of uterine sarcomas
- Subtypes: benign stromal nodules, low grade stromal sarcomas, high grade stromal sarcomas
- Most involve the endometrium with vaginal bleeding
- Diagnosis: uterine curettage

## *Carcinosarcoma (Malignant Mixed Müllerian Tumor)*

- Account for 50% of uterine sarcomas
- Presentation: large polypoid mass filling the endometrial cavity and protruding through the cervical os
- Diagnosis: uterine curettage

## Management

- Initial: total abdominal hysterectomy with bilateral salpingo-oophorectomy, pelvic and paraaortic lymphadenectomy, staging
- Adjuvant therapy
  - Radiation: may decrease local recurrences. May improve local control and prolong survival in carcinosarcomas
  - Chemotherapy
    - Leiomyosarcomas: doxirubicin most active
    - Carcinosarcomas: ifosfamide most active

## SUGGESTED READING

Berek JS, Hacker NF. *Practical gynecologic oncology*, 3rd ed. Philadelphia: Lippincott Williams & Wilkins, 2000.

Rose PG. Medical progress: endometrial cancer. *N Engl J Med* 1996; 335:640–649.

# 83 Vulvar Cancer

*Vulvar cancers often go unrecognized—any suspicious vulvar lesion should be biopsied*

## INTRODUCTION

- 3800 new cases; 800 deaths in 2002
- Mean age at diagnosis: 65

## RISK FACTORS

- **Vulvar intraepithelial neoplasia**
  - Preinvasive vulvar lesion classified as vulvar intraepithelial neoplasia 1–3 based on severity
  - White or red lesion, often raised or papular, may be multifocal
  - Diagnosis: colposcopy with directed biopsy
  - Treatment: wide local excision, superficial vulvectomy, or $CO_2$ laser
- **HPV**
- **Nonneoplastic epithelial disorders of the vulva:** lichen sclerosus
- **Other risk factors:** multiple sex partners, smoking, lymphogranuloma venereum, and granuloma inguinale

## PATHOLOGY

- **Squamous cell carcinoma:** 90% of vulvar carcinomas
- **Melanoma**
  - Most are postmenopausal white women
  - Lesions: pigmented, plaques or nodules
  - Histologic subtypes: superficial spreading, nodular, lentigenous
- **Paget's disease of the vulva**
  - Malignant glandular cells within the epidermis
  - Most are postmenopausal white women
  - Lesions: red, eczematous, sharply demarcated patches
  - 4–8% have associated invasive vulvar adenocarcinoma

- 30% develop synchronous GI, genitourinary, or breast malignancies
- Treatment: local excision
- Increased risk of underlying vulvar adenocarcinoma and other synchronous primary neoplasms
- **Bartholin's gland carcinoma:** 5% of vulvar malignancies
- **Basal cell carcinoma**
  - Arise as ulcers
  - Locally aggressive but metastasis is rare
- **Sarcomas:** rare

## HISTORY

- Vulvar pruritus
- Dysuria
- Vaginal discharge
- Vaginal bleeding

## PHYSICAL EXAM

- Vulvar nodules, ulcers, or plaques
- Lymph node palpation
- Pelvic exam

## DIAGNOSTIC EVALUATION

- Vulvar biopsy
- Cystoscopy, proctoscopy

### Spread

- Most commonly by direct extension
- Lymphatic involvement: first to inguinal then femoral lymph nodes
- Cloquet's node: most cephalad of the femoral nodes
- 25% of patients with groin node involvement have spread to the pelvic lymph nodes

### Staging

- Surgical.
- Staging of melanoma is based on either the level or depth of invasion (Tables 83-1 and 83-2).

## TABLE 83-1.
## STAGING AND SURVIVAL OF NONMELANOMA VULVAR CANCER

| Stage | | 5-yr survival (%) |
|---|---|---|
| I | Tumor <2 cm in diameter, confined to vulva, nodes negative | 98 |
| IA | Stromal invasion <1 mm | |
| IB | Stromal invasion >1 mm | |
| II | Tumor confined to vulva, >2 cm in diameter, nodes negative | 85 |
| III | Tumor of any size with spread to lower urethra, vagina, or anus, or lymph node metastasis | 74 |
| IV | | 31 |
| IVA | Tumor invades bladder mucosa, rectal mucosa, pelvic bone, or bilateral inguinal nodes | |
| IVB | Distant metastasis | |

## MANAGEMENT
### Primary Lesion

- Radical vulvectomy or radical local excision (1-cm margins)
- Large defects may need rhomboid flap or gracilis myocutaneous graft to close

## TABLE 83-2.
## STAGING OF MELANOMA

| | Clark | Chung | Breslow (mm) |
|---|---|---|---|
| I | Intraepithelial | Intraepithelial | <0.76 |
| II | Into papillary dermis | <1 mm from granular layer | 0.76–1.50 |
| III | Filling dermal papillae | 1.1–2.0 mm from granular layer | 1.51–2.25 |
| IV | Into reticular dermis | >2 mm from granular layer | 2.26–3.0 |
| V | Into SC fat | Into subcutaneous fat | >3.0 |

Reprinted from Berek JS, Hacker NF. *Practical gynecologic oncology*, 3rd ed. Philadelphia: Lippincott Williams & Wilkins, 2000:582, with permission.

### Groin Lymph Nodes

- Groin node dissection may be omitted if invasion <1 mm.
- Tumors <2 cm in diameter and >2 cm from midline may undergo unilateral groin dissection.
- All other patients: bilateral inguinofemoral lymphadenectomy.
- Sentinel node mapping is under investigation.

### Adjuvant Therapy

- Positive groin nodes: groin and pelvic irradiation
- Close margins, lymphvascular space involvement; close margins, consider radiation

### Advanced Disease

Preop radiation considered, followed by radical excision or exeneration

### Recurrent Disease

- Local recurrences: radiation or surgical resection
- Distant metastasis: chemotherapy

### Vulvar Melanoma

- Radical local excision for <1 mm of invasion
- Other lesions: radical vulvectomy with bilateral groin node dissection (more conservative treatment most appropriate)
- Adjuvant therapy: interferon alfa-2b (under investigation)

## COMPLICATIONS
### Lymphedema

- Results from removal of normal lymphatic channels
- Initial treatment: physical therapy with elevation of the extremities, exercise
- Compression garments, pneumatic devices help relieve
- Diuretics ineffective

## FOLLOW-UP

- q3mos × 2 yrs, q6mos × 3 yrs, then yearly
- Vulvar exam with acetic acid and colposcopy
- Pap smear and pelvic exam annually

## SUGGESTED READING

Berek JS, Hacker NF. *Practical gynecologic oncology*, 3rd ed. Philadelphia: Lippincott Williams & Wilkins, 2000.

# 84 Gestational Trophoblastic Disease

*Gestational trophoblastic disease is highly curable if recognized early*

## INTRODUCTION

- Gestational trophoblastic neoplasms: tumors derived from placental chorion

- Presentation: hydatiform mole (molar pregnancy) or malignant gestational trophoblastic neoplasia

## HYDATIFORM MOLE
### Pathology

See Table 84-1.

### Clinical Features

- Vaginal bleeding (95%)

- Excessive uterine size (50%)

- Theca lutein cysts (50%)

- Preeclampsia (27%)

- Hyperemesis gravidarum (26%)

- Hyperthyroidism (7%)

- Trophoblastic embolization (2%)

- Partial moles—present as incomplete or missed abortion

### Diagnostic Evaluation

- U/S: snowstorm pattern

- Lab (quantitative beta-hCG, CBC, TSH, electrolytes)

### Management

- Suction curettage. Oxytocin begun before evacuation (bleeding may be heavy).

- Hysterectomy appropriate if childbearing completed.

### Outcome
#### Prognosis

- Complete moles: 15% locally invasive, 4% metastatic

**TABLE 84-1.**
**FEATURES OF COMPLETE AND PARTIAL**
**HYDATIFORM MOLE**

|  | Complete mole | Partial mole |
|---|---|---|
| Karyotype | 46 XX, 46 XY | 69 XXY, 69 XYY |
| Fetal tissue | None | Present |
| Chorionic villi swelling | Diffuse | Focal |
| Trophoblastic hyperplasia | Diffuse | Focal |

- Partial moles: 2–4% locally invasive

### High-Risk Features
hCG >100,000, excessive uterine enlargement, theca lutein cysts >6 cm

### Follow-Up
- hCG weekly until normal for 3 consecutive wks, then monthly until normal for 6 mos
- Hormonal contraception provided

## PERSISTENT GESTATIONAL TROPHOBLASTIC NEOPLASIA
### Introduction
- Arises after molar pregnancy, normal pregnancy, abortion
- Locally invasive or metastatic
- Pathology
- **Invasive mole:** hydropic villi invading myometrium
- **Choriocarcinoma:** proliferating cytotrophoblasts and synctiotrophoblasts, no chorionic villi present
- **Placental site trophoblastic tumor:** intermediate trophoblasts invading myometrium
  - Relatively resistant to chemotherapy
  - hCG often normal, human placental lactogen elevated
  - Treatment: hysterectomy

### History
Vaginal bleeding, cough, hemoptysis, right upper quadrant pain

### Diagnostic Evaluation
- Metastasis: pulmonary (80%), vagina (30%), liver (10%), CNS (10%)

## TABLE 84-2.
## WHO PROGNOSTIC SCORING SYSTEM

| | 0 | 1 | 2 | 4 |
|---|---|---|---|---|
| Age | <39 | >39 | — | — |
| Antecedent pregnancy | Hydatiform mole | Abortion | Term | — |
| Interval between end of antecedent pregnancy and start of chemotherapy (months) | <4 | 4–6 | 7–12 | >12 |
| Human chorionic gonadotropin | $<10^3$ | $10^3–10^4$ | $10^4–10^5$ | $>10^5$ |
| ABO groups | — | O or A | B or AB | — |
| Largest tumor, including uterine (cm) | <3 | 3–5 | >5 | — |
| Site of metastases | — | Spleen, kidney | GI, liver | Brain |
| Number of metastases | — | 1–3 | 4–8 | >8 |
| Prior chemotherapy | — | | 1 drug | >2 drugs |

Reprinted from Bagashwe KD. Treatment of high-risk choriocarcinoma. *J Reprod Med* 1984;29:813, with permission.

- Lab: hCG, liver function tests, CBC, TSH, electrolytes
- Imaging: pelvic U/S; head, chest, and abdominal CT (metastasis)

### *Staging*

- **WHO Prognostic Scoring System:** high risk (score >8), middle risk (5–7), low risk (score <4) categories (Table 84-2) [1]
- **Clinical staging system:** based on prognostic factors (Table 84-3)

## TABLE 84-3.
## CLINICAL STAGING SYSTEM FOR GESTATIONAL TROPHOBLASTIC DISEASE

| Good prognosis | Poor prognosis |
|---|---|
| 1. Pretreatment hCG < 40,000 mIU/mL | 1. Pretreatment hCG > 40,000 mIU/mL |
| 2. No prior chemotherapy | 2. Failure of previous chemotherapy |
| 3. Short duration (<4 mos) | 3. Long duration (>4 mos) |
| | 4. Metastasis to brain, liver |
| | 5. Antecedent term pregnancy |

## TABLE 84-4.
## MANAGEMENT OF GESTATIONAL
## TROPHOBLASTIC DISEASE

| | |
|---|---|
| Stage I | Single-agent chemotherapy |
| Stage II, III[a] | |
|   Low risk | Single-agent chemotherapy |
|   High risk | Combination chemotherapy |
| Stage IV | Combination chemotherapy |

Single-agent chemotherapy: methotrexate, actinomycin D if resistant

Combination chemotherapy: etoposide/methotrexate/actinomycin D/cyclo-phosphamide/vincristine

[a]WHO prognostic scoring system or clinical staging.

- **FIGO staging**
  - Stage I: Confined to uterus
  - Stage II: Pelvic and vaginal metastasis
  - Stage III: Pulmonary metastasis
  - Stage IV: Distant metastasis

### Management

See Table 84-4.

### Outcome

#### Prognosis

- Survival: nonmetastatic (approaches 100%), poor prognosis disease (85%)
- Molar pregnancy recurs in 1–1.5% of subsequent pregnancies

#### Follow-Up

- hCG weekly until normal for 3 consecutive wks, then monthly until normal × 12 mos (24 mos in stage IV disease)
- Hormonal contraception provided

### SUGGESTED READING

Berek JS, Hacker NF. *Practical gynecologic oncology*, 3rd ed. Philadelphia: Lippincott Williams & Wilkins, 2000.
Berkowitz RS, Goldstein DP. Chorionic tumors. *N Engl J Med* 1996;335:1740–1748.

### REFERENCE

1. Bagshawe KD. Treatment of high-risk choriocarcinoma. *J Reprod Med* 1984;29:813.

# 85

# Electrolytes

*Electrolyte abnormalities are common in preop patients*

## ELECTROLYTE SOLUTIONS
See Table 85-1.

## POTASSIUM
### Hypokalemia

- Potassium <3.5 mmol/L

- Manifestations: weakness, myalgias, and arrhythmias

- Differential diagnosis: decreased intake, increased transcellular shifts, renal or nonrenal losses

- Management: oral or parenteral replacement

  - 10 mEq of KCl will increase serum potassium 0.05–0.1 mEq/L

  - IV replacement should not exceed 20 mmol/hr

### Hyperkalemia

- Potassium >5 mEq/L.

- Manifestations: ECG changes (peaked T waves, prolonged PR interval, widened QRS complex), ventricular fibrillation, asystole.

- Differential diagnosis shown in Fig. 85-1.

- Management: emergent therapy if ECG changes present (Table 85-2)

## SODIUM
### Hypernatremia

- Sodium >145 mmol/L.

- Manifestations: altered mental status, weakness, focal neural defects, seizures.

- Differential diagnosis shown in Fig. 85-2.

- Differential diagnosis: usually secondary to water deficit (decreased intake or excessive water loss).

- Evaluation: plasma and urine osmolality, urine sodium.

- Management.

### TABLE 85-1.
### COMPOSITION OF COMMON CRYSTALLOID SOLUTIONS

| Solution | Osmolality (mOsm/kg) | Glucose (g/L) | Sodium (mmol/L) | Chloride (mmol/L) |
|---|---|---|---|---|
| $D_5W$ | 278 | 50 | 0 | 0 |
| $D_{10}W$ | 556 | 100 | 0 | 0 |
| $D_{50}W$ | 2778 | 500 | 0 | 0 |
| 0.45% NaCl (half normal saline) | 154 | — | 77 | 77 |
| 0.9% NaCl (normal saline) | 308 | — | 154 | 154 |
| 3% NaCl | 1026 | — | 513 | 513 |
| Lactated Ringer's | 274 | — | 130 | 109 |

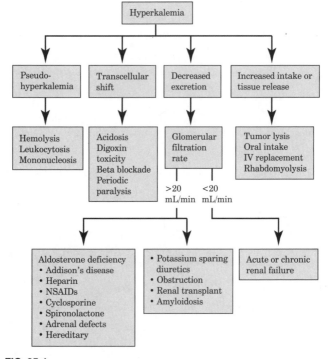

**FIG. 85-1.**
Differential diagnosis of hyperkalemia.

## TABLE 85-2.
## TREATMENT OF HYPERKALEMIA

| Drug | Dose | Onset | Notes |
|------|------|-------|-------|
| Calcium gluconate | 10 mL of 10% solution over 2–3 mins; repeat in 5–10 mins | Minutes<br><br>Lasts only 30–60 mins | Antagonizes potassium at membranes<br><br>Cardioprotective |
| Insulin | 10–20 U regular with 25–50 g glucose | 15–30 mins; lasts hours | Intracellular shift |
| $NaHCO_3$ | 1 ampule IV | 15–30 mins; lasts hours | Intracellular shift<br><br>Reserved for severe metabolic acidosis |
| $Beta_2$-agonists | — | 30 mins; lasts hrs | — |
| Kayexalate | 20–50 g in 100–200 mL 20% sorbitol PO | 1–2 hrs | Cation exchange resin |
| | 50 g in 200 mL 20% sorbitol as enema | Lasts 4–6 hrs | — |
| Dialysis | — | — | Reserved for renal failure and life threatening hyperkalemia |

- Calculate body water deficit (based on normal total body water)
- Body water deficit (L) = [(plasma [Na+] – 140) × total body water in L] / 140
- Total body water = 0.5 × body weight (kg)
- Restore extracellular volume with half normal (0.45%) or quarter normal (0.225%) saline
- Sodium correction should not exceed 0.5 mmol/L/hr (12 mmol/L/d)

### Hyponatremia

- Sodium <135 mmol/L.
- Manifestations: cerebral swelling (nausea, malaise, lethargy, confusion, seizures).
- Differential diagnosis is shown in Fig. 85-3.

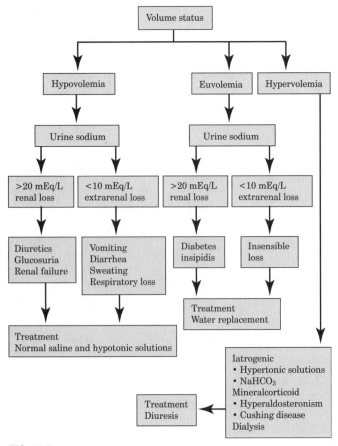

**FIG. 85-2.**
Differential diagnosis of hypernatremia. (Adapted from Prakash UBS, Habermann TM. *Mayo internal medicine board review 2000–2001*. Philadelphia: Lippincott Williams & Wilkins 2000:629.)

- Management.

  - Calculate sodium deficit based on total body water

  - Sodium deficit (mmol) = (130 – current sodium) × total body water

  - Total body water = 0.5 × body weight (kg)

  - After sodium deficit calculated amount of saline (0.9%, 3%) needed to correct is estimated

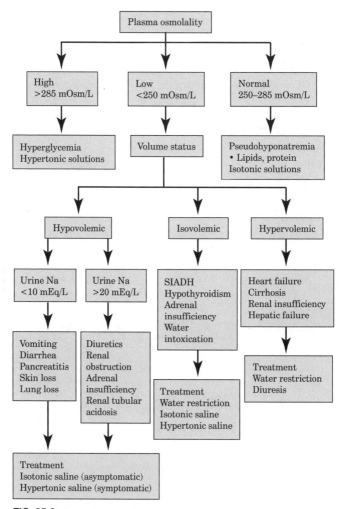

**FIG. 85-3.**
Differential diagnosis of hyponatremia. (Adapted from Prakash UBS, Habermann TM. *Mayo internal medicine board review 2000–2001*. Philadelphia: Lippincott Williams & Wilkins 2000:629.)

- Maximum rate of sodium correction should not exceed 0.5 mEq/L/hr.
  - Determine how many hours needed to replace sodium
  - Too rapid correction results in central pontine myelinolysis.

## CALCIUM
### Hypercalcemia

- Manifestations: usually occur if calcium >12 mg/dL
  - Renal (polyuria, nephrolithiasis)
  - GI (anorexia, nausea and vomiting, constipation, ileus)
  - Neurologic (weakness, fatigue, confusion, stupor, coma)
  - Cardiac (ECG with shortened QT interval)
- Evaluation
  - Calcium, ionized calcium, albumin, and PTH measured
  - Calcium corrected for hypoalbuminemia
- Total serum calcium = [(normal albumin – patient albumin) × 0.8] + measured calcium
- Differential diagnosis is listed in Table 85-3.
- Management
  - Initial: extracellular fluid replacement with saline diuresis.

**TABLE 85-3.**
**DIFFERENTIAL DIAGNOSIS OF HYPERCALCEMIA**

Primary hyperparathyroidism

    Adenoma (85%)

    Hyperplasia (15%)

    Parathyroid carcinoma (<1%)

Malignancy

    Osteolytic

    Humoral (PTH-related peptide)

Sarcoidosis

Vitamin D toxicity

Hyperthyroidism

Milk-alkali syndrome

Immobilization

Thiazide diuretics

Familial hypocalciuric hypercalcemia

## TABLE 85-4.
## TREATMENT OF HYPERCALCEMIA

| Treatment | Dose | Onset | Notes |
|---|---|---|---|
| NS | 300–500 mL/hr; 3–4 L in 24 hrs | — | Obtain urine output of 100–200 mL/hr |
| Furosemide | 20–40 mg IV bid–qid | — | Not given unless evidence of heart failure develops |
| Pamidronate | 60 mg in 500 mL NS over 4 hrs; one-time dose | 2 d | — |
| | 90 mg if calcium >13.5 mg/dL | Last 2 wks | — |
| Calcitonin | 4–8 IU/kg IM or SC q6–12h | Several hrs | Safe in renal failure / Analgesic effect if skeletal metastasis / Less potent than pamidronate |
| Plicamycin | 25 g/kg in 500 mL $D_5W$ over 4–6 hrs | 2–4 d | Second line / Thrombocytopenia, renal and liver dysfunction |
| Prednisone | 25–50 mg PO bid | 5–10 d | — |
| Dialysis | — | — | Use if CHF, renal insufficiency |

- Pamidronate or another inhibitor of bone resorption should be given early.
- See Table 85-4.

## SUGGESTED READING

Ahya SN, Flood K, Paranjothi S. *The Washington manual of medical therapeutics*, 30th ed. Philadelphia: Lippincott Williams & Wilkins, 2001.

Fauci AS, et al. *Harrison's principles of internal medicine*, 15th ed. New York: McGraw-Hill, 2001.

Prakash UBS, Habermann TM. *Mayo internal medicine board review 2000–2001*. Philadelphia: Lippincott Williams & Wilkins, 2000.

# Appendixes

# Critical Care

## INTRODUCTION

- Pulmonary artery wedge pressure is a measure of LV preload.

- Obtained by placement of Swan-Ganz catheter.

- Normal hemodynamic parameters are shown in Table A-1.

**TABLE A-1.**
**NORMAL HEMODYNAMIC PARAMETERS**

| Parameter | Formula | Normal value |
| --- | --- | --- |
| Mean arterial pressure | [Systolic arterial pressure + (2 × diastolic pressure)] / 3 | 70–100 mm Hg |
| Pulmonary artery pressure | | 15–30/5–13 mm Hg |
| Central venous pressure | | 5–10 mm Hg |
| Pulmonary capillary wedge pressure | | 2–12 mm Hg |
| Stroke volume | | 60–120 mL/contraction |
| Cardiac output | Stroke volume × heart rate | 3–7 L/min |
| Cardiac index | Cardiac output / body surface area | 2.5–4.5 L/min/m$^2$ |
| Systemic vascular resistance | | 800–1200 dynes/sec/cm$^{-5}$ |
| Pulmonary vascular resistance | | 120–250 dynes/sec/cm$^{-5}$ |

# Blood Component Therapy

## TABLE B-1.
## BLOOD COMPONENT THERAPY

| Component | Volume | Contents | Effect |
|---|---|---|---|
| Packed RBCs | 200–250 mL | Erythrocytes | Increase Hgb 1 g/dL and Hct 1–3% |
| Platelets | 40 mL | Platelets | Increase platelet count 5000–10,000/mm$^3$ |
| Fresh frozen plasma | 200–250 mL | Clotting factors | Increases clotting factors by 2–3% |
| Cryoprecipitate | 10–15 mL | Factor VIII, XIII, von Willebrand factor, fibrinogen, fibronectin | Increase fibrinogen by 150 mg/U |

# Acid-Base Disorders

## INTRODUCTION

- Acidemia: decreased bicarbonate ($HCO_3^-$) or increased carbon dioxide ($PCO_2$).

- Alkalemia: increased $HCO_3^-$ or decreased $PCO_2$.

- Primary and compensatory responses are shown in Table C-1.

- Differential diagnosis shown in Table C-2.

## MANAGEMENT
### Metabolic Acidosis

- Treat underlying cause.

- If pH <7.20, consider administering parenteral $NaHCO_3$.

### Metabolic Alkalosis

- Treat underlying cause.

- Most commonly caused by vomiting or diuretic use.

- Correct hypovolemia, hypokalemia, hypomagnesemia.

### Respiratory Acidosis

- Treat underlying cause.

- Usually secondary to hypoventilation.

- Ventilatory assistance may be required.

### Respiratory Alkalosis

Secondary to hyperventilation.

## TABLE C-1.
## PRIMARY AND COMPENSATORY RESPONSES IN
## ACID-BASE DISORDERS

Approach to ABGs

1. Examine the pH: acidosis or alkalosis

   Examine [$HCO_3^-$]. In primary metabolic disorders it moves the same direction as pH.

   Examine the $PCO_2$. In primary respiratory disorders it moves the opposite direction of pH.

2. Is there adequate compensation?

3. If metabolic acidosis is present, calculate the anion gap.

   Anion gap = $(Na^+ + K^+) - Cl^-$

   Normal anion gap is $10^{-14}$

| Disorder | Primary change | Compensatory response |
|---|---|---|
| Metabolic acidosis | ↓ [$HCO_3^-$] | ↓ $PCO_2$ by 1.0–1.3 mm Hg for every 1 mmol/L ↓ [$HCO_3^-$] |
| | | $PCO_2$ should equal last 2 digits of pH × 100 |
| Metabolic alkalosis | ↑ [$HCO_3^-$] | ↑ $PCO_2$ 0.6–0.7 mm Hg for every 1 mmol/L ↑ [$HCO_3^-$] |
| Respiratory acidosis | ↑ $PCO_2$ | |
| Acute | | ↑ [$HCO_3^-$] 1 mmol/L for every 10 mm Hg ↑ $PCO_2$ |
| Chronic | | ↑ [$HCO_3^-$] 3.0–3.5 mmol/L for every 10 mm Hg ↑ $PCO_2$ |
| Respiratory alkalosis | ↓ $PCO_2$ | |
| Acute | | ↓ [$HCO_3^-$] 2 mmol/L for every 10 mm Hg ↓ $PCO_2$ |
| Chronic | | ↓ [$HCO_3^-$] 4–5 mmol/L for every 10 mm Hg ↓ $PCO_2$ (pH usually normal range) |

Reprinted from Ahya SN, Flood K, Paranjothi S. *The Washington manual of medical therapeutics*, 30th ed. Philadelphia: Lippincott Williams & Wilkins, 2001:70, with permission.

## TABLE C-2.
## DIFFERENTIAL DIAGNOSIS OF ACID-BASE DISORDERS

| | |
|---|---|
| Metabolic acidosis | Increased anion gap |
| |     Uremia |
| |     Ketoacidosis (diabetes, ethanol) |
| |     Salicylates |
| |     Ethylene glycol |
| |     Lactic acidosis |
| |     Methanol |
| |     Paraldehyde |
| | Normal anion gap |
| |     GI loss (diarrhea, urinary diversion) |
| |     Exogenous acid |
| |     Proximal (type 2) renal tubular acidosis |
| |     Hyperkalemic (type 4) renal tubular acidosis |
| |     Drugs (potassium-sparing diuretics, ACE inhibitors, NSAIDs, TMP) |
| |     Renal insufficiency |
| |     Rapid saline infusion |
| |     Classic distal (type 1) renal tubular acidosis |
| Metabolic alkalosis | Chloride responsive (urine chloride <10 mmol/L) |
| | GI (vomiting, NG suction, cystic fibrosis) |
| | Renal (diuretics, posthypercapnic state, nonreabsorbable anions) |
| | Exogenous alkali (antacids, massive transfusion) |
| | Contraction alkalosis |
| | Chloride unresponsive (urine chloride >10 mmol/L) |
| | Potassium or magnesium depletion |
| | Bartter's syndrome |
| | Hypercalcemia |
| | Hypertensive (primary aldosteronism, Cushing's syndrome, exogenous mineralcorticoid, pseudohyperaldosteronism) |
| Respiratory acidosis | Central respiratory depression (drugs, sleep apnea, obesity, CNS disease) |

*(continued)*

## TABLE C-2.
## CONTINUED

|  | Airway obstruction (foreign body, bronchospasm) |
|---|---|
|  | Neuromuscular disease (polio, kyphoscoliosis, myasthenia) |
|  | Parenchymal lung disease (COPD, pneumothorax, pneumonia, pulmonary edema, interstitial lung disease) |
| Respiratory alkalosis | Central stimulation (anxiety, pain, head trauma, cerebrovascular accident, fever, salicylates, thyroxine, progesterone) |
|  | Hypoxemia |
|  | Airway irritation |
|  | Pulmonary embolism |
|  | Hepatic failure |
|  | Pregnancy |
|  | Hyperthyroidism |

## SUGGESTED READING

Ahya SN, Flood K, Paranjothi S. *The Washington manual of medical therapeutics*, 30th ed. Philadelphia: Lippincott Williams & Wilkins, 2001.

# Lab Reference Values

Tables D-1, D-2, and D-3 list commonly used lab reference values. The values are those currently used by the Barnes-Jewish Hospital.

## TABLE D-1.
## SERUM CHEMISTRIES

| | |
|---|---|
| Aminotransferases | |
| ALT | 7–53 IU/L |
| AST | 11–47 IU/L |
| Albumin | 3.6–5.0 g/dL |
| Blood gas | |
| pH | 7.35–7.45 |
| $P_{CO_2}$ | 80–105 mm Hg |
| $P_{O_2}$ | 35–45 mm Hg |
| Calcium | |
| Total | 8.6–10.3 mg/dL |
| Ionized | 4.5–5.1 mg/dL |
| Ferritin (adult female) | 10–283 ng/mL |
| Hgb A1C | 4.0–6.0% |
| Iron (female) | 30–160 µg/dL |
| Folate | |
| Plasma | 3.1–12.4 ng/mL |
| Red cell | 186–645 ng/mL |
| Iron-binding capacity | 220–420 µg/dL |
| Troponin I | |
| Normal | <0.6 ng/mL |
| Indeterminant | 0.7–1.4 ng/mL |
| Abnormal | >1.5 ng/mL |
| Lactate | 0.7–2.1 mmol/L |
| Uric acid | 3–8 mg/dL |
| Transferrin saturation | 20–50% |

## TABLE D-2.
## SERUM HORMONE LEVELS

| | |
|---|---|
| ACTH (fasting, 8 A.M.) | <60 pg/mL |
| Cortisol (Plasma, A.M.) | 6–30 mg/dL |
| FSH | |
|     Follicular | 4–13 IU/L |
|     Luteal | 2–13 IU/L |
|     Midcycle | 5–22 IU/L |
|     Postmenopausal | 20–138 IU/L |
| Growth hormone (fast) | <10 ng/mL |
| 17-Hydroxyprogesterone | |
|     Follicular | <80 ng/dL |
|     Luteal | <235 ng/dL |
|     Postmenopausal | <51 ng/dL |
| Insulin (fasting) | 3–15 mU/L |
| LH | |
|     Follicular | 1–18 IU/L |
|     Luteal | <20 IU/L |
|     Midcycle | 24–105 IU/L |
|     Postmenopausal | 15–62 IU/L |
| Prolactin | 1.4–24.2 ng/mL |
| Progesterone | |
|     Follicular | 0.1–1.5 ng/mL |
|     Luteal | 2.5–28.0 ng/mL |
|     First trimester | 9–47 ng/mL |
|     Third trimester | 55–255 ng/mL |
|     Postmenopausal | <0.5 ng/mL |
| Testosterone | |
|     Total | 6–86 ng/dL |
|     Free | 0.3–1.9 ng/dL |
| Thyroxine | |
|     Total | 4.5–12.0 µg/dL |
|     Free | 0.7–1.8 ng/dL |
| TSH | 0.35–6.20 mU/mL |

## TABLE D-3.
## ANTIMICROBIALS

| | |
|---|---|
| Gentamycin | |
| Peak | 6–10 mg/L |
| Trough | 0.5–2.0 mg/L |
| Tobramycin | |
| Peak | 6–10 mg/L |
| Trough | 0.5–2.0 mg/L |
| Vancomycin | |
| Peak | 20–40 mg/L |
| Trough | 5–15 mg/L |

# Ultrasound Tables

**TABLE E-1.**
**PREDICTED MENSTRUAL AGE FOR CROWN–RUMP LENGTH**

| CRL | MA | CRL | MA | CRL | MA | CRL | MA | CRL | MA | CRL | MA |
|-----|-----|-----|------|-----|------|-----|------|------|------|------|------|
| 0.2 | 5.7 | 2.2 | 8.9  | 4.2 | 11.1 | 6.2 | 12.6 | 8.2  | 14.2 | 10.2 | 16.1 |
| 0.3 | 5.9 | 2.3 | 9.0  | 4.3 | 11.2 | 6.3 | 12.7 | 8.3  | 14.2 | 10.3 | 16.2 |
| 0.4 | 6.1 | 2.4 | 9.1  | 4.4 | 11.2 | 6.4 | 128  | 8.4  | 14.3 | 10.4 | 16.3 |
| 0.5 | 6.2 | 2.5 | 9.2  | 4.5 | 11.3 | 6.5 | 12.8 | 8.5  | 14.4 | 10.5 | 16.4 |
| 0.6 | 6.4 | 2.6 | 9.4  | 4.6 | 11.4 | 6.6 | 12.9 | 8.6  | 14.5 | 10.6 | 16.5 |
| 0.7 | 6.6 | 2.7 | 9.5  | 4.7 | 11.5 | 6.7 | 13.0 | 8.7  | 14.6 | 10.7 | 16.6 |
| 0.8 | 6.7 | 2.8 | 9.6  | 4.8 | 11.6 | 6.8 | 13.1 | 8.8  | 14.7 | 10.8 | 16.7 |
| 0.9 | 6.9 | 2.9 | 9.7  | 4.9 | 11.7 | 6.9 | 13.1 | 8.9  | 14.8 | 10.9 | 16.8 |
| 1.0 | 7.2 | 3.0 | 9.9  | 5.0 | 11.7 | 7.0 | 13.2 | 9.0  | 14.9 | 11.0 | 16.9 |
| 1.1 | 7.2 | 3.1 | 10.0 | 5.1 | 11.8 | 7.1 | 13.3 | 9.1  | 15.0 | 11.1 | 17.0 |
| 1.2 | 7.4 | 3.2 | 10.1 | 5.2 | 11.9 | 7.2 | 13.4 | 9.2  | 15.1 | 11.2 | 17.1 |
| 1.3 | 7.5 | 3.3 | 10.2 | 5.3 | 12.0 | 7.3 | 13.4 | 9.3  | 15.2 | 11.3 | 17.2 |
| 1.4 | 7.7 | 3.4 | 10.3 | 5.4 | 12.0 | 7.4 | 13.5 | 9.4  | 15.3 | 11.4 | 17.3 |
| 1.5 | 7.9 | 3.5 | 10.4 | 5.5 | 12.1 | 7.5 | 13.6 | 9.5  | 15.3 | 11.5 | 17.4 |
| 1.6 | 8.0 | 3.6 | 10.5 | 5.6 | 12.2 | 7.6 | 13.7 | 9.6  | 15.4 | 11.6 | 17.5 |
| 1.7 | 8.1 | 3.7 | 10.6 | 5.7 | 12.3 | 7.7 | 13.8 | 9.7  | 15.5 | 11.7 | 17.6 |
| 1.8 | 8.3 | 3.8 | 10.7 | 5.8 | 12.3 | 7.8 | 13.8 | 9.8  | 15.6 | 11.8 | 17.7 |
| 1.9 | 8.4 | 3.9 | 10.8 | 5.9 | 12.4 | 7.9 | 13.9 | 9.9  | 15.7 | 11.9 | 17.8 |
| 2.0 | 8.6 | 4.0 | 10.9 | 6.0 | 12.5 | 8.0 | 14.0 | 10.0 | 15.9 | 12.0 | 17.9 |
| 2.1 | 8.7 | 4.1 | 11.0 | 6.1 | 12.6 | 8.1 | 14.1 | 10.1 | 16.0 | 12.1 | 18.0 |

CRL, crown–rump length (cm); MA, menstrual age (wks).
Adapted from Hadlock FP, Shah YP, Kanon DJ, Lindsey JV. Fetal crown-rump length: Reevaluation of relation to menstrual age (5–18 wks) with high resolution real-time US. *Radiology* 1992;182:501–505.

**TABLE E-2.**
**MEAN SAC DIAMETER, MENSTRUAL AGE, AND HCG**

| Menstrual age (wks) | hCG reference range (mIU/mL) |
| --- | --- |
| Nonpregnant female | <5 |
| 3–4 | 9–130 |
| 4–5 | 75–2600 |
| 5–6 | 850–20,800 |
| 6–7 | 4000–100,200 |
| 7–12 | 11,500–289,000 |
| 12–16 | 18,300–137,000 |
| 16–29 | 1400–53,000 |
| 29–41 | 940–60,000 |

## TABLE E-3.
## PREDICTED MENSTRUAL AGE FOR HEAD CIRCUMFERENCE MEASUREMENTS

| Head circumference (cm) | Menstrual age (wks) | Head circumference (cm) | Menstrual age (wks) |
|---|---|---|---|
| 8.5 | 13.7 | 22.5 | 24.4 |
| 9.0 | 14.0 | 23.0 | 24.9 |
| 9.5 | 14.3 | 23.5 | 25.4 |
| 10.0 | 14.6 | 24.0 | 25.9 |
| 10.5 | 15.0 | 24.5 | 26.4 |
| 11.0 | 15.3 | 52.0 | 26.9 |
| 11.5 | 15.6 | 25.5 | 27.5 |
| 12.0 | 15.9 | 26.0 | 28.6 |
| 12.5 | 16.3 | 26.5 | 28.6 |
| 13.0 | 16.6 | 27.0 | 29.2 |
| 13.5 | 17.0 | 27.5 | 29.8 |
| 14.0 | 17.3 | 28.0 | 30.3 |
| 14.5 | 17.7 | 28.5 | 31.0 |
| 15.0 | 18.1 | 29.0 | 31.6 |
| 15.5 | 18.4 | 29.5 | 32.2 |
| 16.0 | 18.8 | 30.0 | 32.8 |
| 16.5 | 19.2 | 30.5 | 33.5 |
| 17.0 | 19.6 | 31.0 | 34.2 |
| 17.5 | 20.0 | 31.5 | 34.9 |
| 18.0 | 20.4 | 32.0 | 35.5 |
| 18.5 | 20.8 | 32.5 | 36.3 |
| 19.0 | 21.2 | 33.0 | 37.0 |
| 19.5 | 21.6 | 33.5 | 37.7 |
| 20.0 | 22.1 | 34.0 | 38.5 |
| 20.5 | 22.5 | 34.5 | 39.2 |
| 21.0 | 23.0 | 35.0 | 40.0 |
| 21.5 | 23.4 | 35.5 | 40.8 |
| 22.0 | 23.9 | 36.0 | 41.6 |

Adapted from Hadlock FP, Deter RL, Harrist RB, Park SK. Fetal head circumference: Relation to menstrual age. *AJR Am J Roentgenol* 1982;138:649.

## TABLE E-4.
## PREDICTED MENSTRUAL AGE FOR ABDOMINAL CIRCUMFERENCE MEASUREMENTS

| Abdominal circumference (cm) | Menstrual age (wks) | Abdominal circumference (cm) | Menstrual age (wks) |
|---|---|---|---|
| 10.0 | 15.6 | 23.5 | 27.7 |
| 10.5 | 16.1 | 24.0 | 28.2 |
| 11.0 | 16.5 | 24.5 | 28.7 |
| 11.5 | 16.9 | 52.0 | 29.2 |
| 12.0 | 17.3 | 25.5 | 29.7 |
| 12.5 | 17.8 | 26.0 | 30.1 |
| 13.0 | 18.2 | 26.5 | 30.6 |
| 13.5 | 18.6 | 27.0 | 31.1 |
| 14.0 | 19.1 | 27.5 | 31.6 |
| 14.5 | 19.5 | 28.0 | 32.1 |
| 15.0 | 20.0 | 28.5 | 32.6 |
| 15.5 | 20.4 | 29.0 | 33.1 |
| 16.0 | 20.8 | 29.5 | 33.6 |
| 16.5 | 21.3 | 30.0 | 34.1 |
| 17.0 | 21.7 | 30.5 | 34.6 |
| 17.5 | 22.2 | 31.0 | 35.1 |
| 18.0 | 22.6 | 31.5 | 35.6 |
| 18.5 | 23.1 | 32.0 | 36.1 |
| 19.0 | 23.6 | 32.5 | 36.6 |
| 19.5 | 24.0 | 33.0 | 37.1 |
| 20.0 | 24.5 | 33.5 | 37.6 |
| 20.5 | 24.9 | 34.0 | 38.1 |
| 21.0 | 25.4 | 34.5 | 38.7 |
| 21.5 | 25.9 | 35.0 | 39.2 |
| 22.0 | 26.3 | 35.5 | 39.7 |
| 22.5 | 26.8 | 36.0 | 40.2 |
| 23.0 | 27.3 | | |

Adapted from Hadlock FP, Deter RL, Harrist RB, Park SK. Fetal abdominal circumference as a predictor of menstrual age. *AJR Am J Roentgenol* 1982; 139:367.

## TABLE E-5.
## PREDICTED MENSTRUAL AGE FOR FEMUR
## LENGTH MEASUREMENTS

| Femur length (cm) | Menstrual age (wks) | Femur length (cm) | Menstrual age (wks) |
|---|---|---|---|
| 1.0 | 12.8 | 4.5 | 24.5 |
| 1.1 | 13.1 | 4.6 | 24.9 |
| 1.2 | 13.4 | 4.7 | 25.3 |
| 1.3 | 13.6 | 4.8 | 25.7 |
| 1.4 | 13.9 | 4.9 | 26.1 |
| 1.5 | 14.2 | 5.0 | 26.5 |
| 1.6 | 14.5 | 5.1 | 27.0 |
| 1.7 | 14.8 | 5.2 | 27.4 |
| 1.8 | 15.1 | 5.3 | 27.8 |
| 1.9 | 15.4 | 5.4 | 28.2 |
| 2.0 | 15.7 | 5.5 | 28.7 |
| 2.1 | 16.0 | 5.6 | 29.1 |
| 2.2 | 16.3 | 5.7 | 29.6 |
| 2.3 | 16.6 | 5.8 | 30.0 |
| 2.4 | 16.9 | 5.9 | 30.8 |
| 2.5 | 17.2 | 6.0 | 30.9 |
| 2.6 | 17.6 | 6.1 | 31.4 |
| 2.7 | 17.9 | 6.2 | 31.9 |
| 2.8 | 18.2 | 6.3 | 32.3 |
| 2.9 | 18.6 | 6.4 | 32.8 |
| 3.0 | 18.9 | 6.5 | 33.3 |
| 3.1 | 19.2 | 6.6 | 33.8 |
| 3.2 | 19.6 | 6.7 | 34.2 |
| 3.3 | 19.9 | 6.8 | 34.7 |
| 3.4 | 20.3 | 6.9 | 35.2 |
| 3.5 | 20.7 | 7.0 | 35.7 |
| 3.6 | 21.0 | 7.1 | 36.2 |
| 3.7 | 21.4 | 7.2 | 36.7 |
| 3.8 | 21.8 | 7.3 | 37.2 |
| 3.9 | 22.1 | 7.4 | 37.7 |
| 4.0 | 22.5 | 7.5 | 38.3 |
| 4.1 | 22.9 | 7.6 | 38.8 |
| 4.2 | 23.3 | 7.7 | 39.3 |
| 4.3 | 23.7 | 7.8 | 39.8 |
| 4.4 | 24.1 | 7.9 | 40.4 |

Adapted from Hadlock FP, Deter RL, Harrist RB, Park SK. Fetal femur length as a predictor of menstrual age: sonographically measured. *AJR Am J Roentgenol* 1982;138:875.

# Anticoagulation

Tables F-1 and F-2 are based on anticoagulation guidelines developed by the Barnes-Jewish Hospital.

### TABLE F-1.
### HEPARIN NOMOGRAM

| | | |
|---|---|---|
| Initial bolus | 60 U/kg (max, 5000 U) | |
| Initial infusion rate | 14 U/kg/hr | |
| Draw STAT PTT 6 hrs after bolus | | |
|     PTT 45–70 | None | No change |
|     PTT 71–80 | None | Decrease 1 U/kg/hr |
|     PTT 81–90 | Hold 30 mins | Decrease 2 U/kg/hr |
|     PTT >90 | Hold 1 hr | Decrease 3 U/kg/hr |
| Draw STAT PTT 6 hrs after each rate change. After 2 consecutive PTTs are therapeutic (45–70 secs) draw PTT qam | | |

## TABLE F-2.
## TREATMENT OF WARFARIN-INDUCED BLEEDING

| | |
|---|---|
| INR >5; no bleeding | Hold warfarin |
| | Search for occult bleed |
| | Evaluate drug interactions |
| | Follow INR |
| INR 7–10; no bleeding | Vitamin K, 1–2.5 mg PO |
| | Document fall in INR (within 24 hrs of vitamin K) |
| | Redose vitamin K if INR remains high |
| INR >10; no bleeding | Admit patient |
| | Vitamin K, 3 mg SC |
| | Follow INR q6–8h and repeat vitamin K as necessary |
| Minor bleeding | Hold warfarin |
| | Vitamin K, 1–5 mg SC |
| | Follow INR q6–24h and repeat vitamin K prn |
| | If bleeding uncontrolled, treat as major bleeding |
| Major bleeding | Admit patient |
| | Hold warfarin |
| | Vitamin K, 10 mg SC or 10 mg IVPB over 30 mins and fresh frozen plasma |
| | Follow INR q6–24h and repeat vitamin K until INR normal |
| | Control bleed |

## TABLE F-3.
## ACOG CONDITIONS FOR ADJUSTED-DOSE HEPARIN PROPHYLAXIS DURING PREGNANCY

Artificial heart valve

Antithrombin III deficiency

Antiphospholipid antibody syndrome

History of rheumatic heart disease with atrial fibrillation

Homozygous factor V Leiden mutation

Homozygous prothrombin G20210A

Recurrent thromboembolism

**TABLE F-4.**
**ACOG LOW-DOSE AND ADJUSTED-DOSE PROPHYLACTIC
HEPARIN REGIMENS IN PREGNANCY**

| | |
|---|---|
| Low-dose unfractionated heparin | |
| First trimester | 5000–7000 U q12h |
| Second trimester | 7500–10,000 U q12h |
| Third trimester | 10,000 U q12h (unless PTT elevated) |
| Low-dose unfractionated heparin | 5000–10,000 U q12h |
| Adjusted-dose unfractionated heparin prophylaxis | >10,000 U bid–tid to achieve PTT 1.5–2.5 |
| LMWH low-dose prophylaxis | Dalteparin, 5000 U qd or bid |
| | Enoxaparin 40 mg qd or bid |
| LMWH adjusted-dose prophylaxis | Dalteparin, 5000–10,000 U q12h |
| | Enoxaparin, 30–80 mg q12h |

Adapted from the American College of Obstetricians and Gynecologists.
*Thromboembolism in pregnancy. ACOG Practice Bulletin 19*. Washington,
DC: ACOG, 2000.

# G

# Methotrexate Protocol

The following is the Washington University Division of Reproductive Endocrinology protocol for the administration of methotrexate for ectopic pregnancy.

## CRITERIA

The following criteria must be met:

- Mass <3.5 cm
- Unruptured
- Minimal symptoms
- No fetal heart tones
- Stable vital signs

## CONSENT

Obtain informed consent and place on the chart.

## LAB

### Day 1 (Methotrexate Administered)

- Quantitative hCG
- Liver function tests, BUN, creatinine
- CBC
- Type and screen (RhoGAM if Rh negative)

### Day 4

Quantitative hCG

### Day 7 and Weekly

Quantitative hCG until hCG is <2. If there is a <15% decline in hCG or a rise between days 4 and 7, then a repeat dose of methotrexate is given or surgery is considered.

## ADMINISTRATION

1. Obtain height and weight and calculate body surface area (BSA).
2. Calculate dose by multiplying 50 mg/m$^2$ × BSA.

- Example: if the patient was 60 in. tall and weighed 118 lbs, her BSA is 1.5 $m^2$. Therefore 50 mg/$m^2$ × 1.5 $m^2$ = 75 mg of methotrexate.
- Max. dose of methotrexate is 1.5 g.

3. Write an order for methotrexate to be prepared under biological containment hood to be ready for IM injection in 2 syringes. Half of the total dose should be placed in each syringe.
4. Administer dose as IM injections, 1 syringe in each hip.

## FOLLOW-UP

1. Counsel patient about contraception. Before hCG drops <2, barrier methods are used. After hCG drops to 2, hormonal contraception may be initiated.
2. Repeat U/S if pain increased.
3. Counsel patient that she is at increased risk for future ectopic pregnancy.

# Barnes-Jewish Hospital at Washington University Medical Center Antibiogram

**TABLE H.1**
**PERCENTAGE (%) GRAM-POSITIVE STRAINS SUSCEPTIBLE**

| Gram-positive cocci | No. of strains | Oxacillin (cefazolin) | Tetra-cycline | Clinda-mycin | Nitro-furantoin | Erythro-mycin | Cipro-floxacin | TMP/ SMX | Genta-mycin | Peni-cillin | Ceftri-axone | Cefe-pime | Ampi-cillin | High-level strep | High-level gent | Vanco-mycin |
|---|---|---|---|---|---|---|---|---|---|---|---|---|---|---|---|---|
| S. aureus | 2941 | 52 | — | 55 | — | 40 | 48 | 89 | 86 | 7 | — | — | — | — | — | 100 |
| Staphylococcus species not S. aureus | 1215 | 28 | — | 67 | — | 29 | 45 | 50 | 80 | 7 | — | — | — | — | — | 100 |
| E. faecalis | 356 | — | 40 | — | 99 | — | 12 | — | — | — | — | — | 99 | 67 | 62 | 93 |
| E. faecium | 238 | — | 46 | — | 57 | — | 1 | — | — | — | — | — | 11 | 18 | 64 | 21 |
| S. pneumoniae | 183 | — | — | — | — | 77 | — | — | — | 63 | 84 | 72 | — | — | — | — |

# TABLE H.2
## PERCENTAGE (%) GRAM-NEGATIVE STRAINS SUSCEPTIBLE

| Gram-negative cocci | No. of strains | Ampicillin | Cefazolin | Cefotetan | Ceftriaxone | Cefepime | Piperacillin-tazobactam | Imipenem | Gentamycin | Tobramycin | TMP/SMX | Ciprofloxacin |
|---|---|---|---|---|---|---|---|---|---|---|---|---|
| A. baumanii | 174 | — | — | — | 1 | 60 | 44 | 100 | 73 | 95 | 61 | — |
| C. freundii | 97 | 0 | 0 | 60 | 74 | 97 | 80 | 100 | 90 | 74 | 72 | 89 |
| C. koseri | 204 | 0 | 95 | 100 | 98 | 98 | 95 | 100 | 98 | 86 | 99 | 97 |
| E. coli | 4932 | 54 | 89 | 98 | 99 | 99 | 94 | 100 | 98 | 97 | 86 | 97 |
| E. cloacae | 428 | 0 | 0 | 55 | 68 | 93 | 74 | 100 | 96 | 90 | 83 | 86 |
| K. oxytoca | 167 | 0 | 32 | 100 | 82 | 83 | 81 | 100 | 92 | 81 | 87 | 87 |
| K. pneumoniae | 1291 | 0 | 89 | 98 | 95 | 95 | 88 | 100 | 97 | 93 | 83 | 89 |
| M. morganii | 99 | 0 | 0 | 91 | 93 | 100 | 93 | 100 | 93 | 94 | 79 | 80 |
| P. mirabillis | 762 | 90 | 94 | 100 | 99 | 99 | 100 | 100 | 95 | 94 | 89 | 91 |
| P. vulgaris | 15 | 0 | 0 | 100 | 93 | 100 | 100 | 100 | 100 | 100 | 93 | 100 |
| P. aeruginosa | 2087 | — | — | — | 17 | 81 | 87 | 78 | 70 | 81 | — | 59 |
| S. marcescens | 194 | 0 | 0 | 94 | 80 | 95 | 88 | 100 | 89 | 84 | 78 | 79 |
| S. maltophilia | 205 | — | — | — | — | — | — | — | — | — | 86 | — |

# Patient Data Tracking Form

| Name: | |
|---|---|
| DOB | Age |
| Admitted | Discharged |
| Allergies | |

HPI

PMH/PSH

Admission Meds

SH                              FH


ROS

**Admission**

| T | P | R | BP |
|---|---|---|---|
| O2 | | Wt | Ht |

MCV=
RDW=

| Ca | | T bili | | PTT | | | |
|---|---|---|---|---|---|---|---|
| Mg | | D bili | | PT | | | |
| Phos | | AST | | INR | | | |
| TP | | ALT | | Amylase | | | |
| Alb | | Alk Ph | | Lipase | | | |

Previous Labs:

EKG                             CXR

Admission:                      Admission:

Previous:                       Previous:

Previous Studies:

| Admission | Discharge |
|---|---|
| ❏ Old data | ❏ Placement |
| ❏ Old records | |
| ❏ DDx | ❏ Home care |
| ❏ Admit orders | |
| ❏ Interview | ❏ D/C orders |

Problems:

Brief Course

- ❏ H&P
- ❏ Schedule tests
- ❏ Read
- ❏ DVT Proph

- ❏ Transport

| Date | | | | | | | | |
|---|---|---|---|---|---|---|---|---|
| Overnight Complaints | | | | | | | | |
| | CP | | SOB | | CP | | SOB | |
| | N/V | | Abd | | N/V | | Abd | |
| | Urine | | Ap/wt | | Urine | | Ap/wt | |
| | Fatig | | BM | | Fatig | | BM | |
| | HA | | Vis | | HA | | Vis | |
| | Aud | | | | Aud | | | |
| Meds | | | | | | | | |
| Relevant Tests | | | | | | | | |
| T (Tmax) | | | | | | | | |
| P | | | | | | | | |
| R | | | | | | | | |
| BP | | | | | | | | |
| SaO$_2$ | | | | | | | | |
| I/O | | | | | | | | |
| Accu | | | | | | | | |
| Physical Exam | | | | | | | | |

| Other Labs | | | |
|---|---|---|---|
| Tasks | ❏ Pre-round <br> ❏ Notes in chart <br> ❏ Vitals <br> ❏ Meds <br> ❏ Labs <br> ❏ Micro <br> ❏ Note <br> ❏ Order tests <br> ❏ AM Labs | ❏ Change meds <br> ❏ Call consults <br> ❏ Read consults <br><br> ❏ Test results <br> ❏ Chat with pt | ❏ Pre-round <br> ❏ Notes in chart <br> ❏ Vitals <br> ❏ Meds <br> ❏ Labs <br> ❏ Micro <br> ❏ Note <br> ❏ Order tests <br> ❏ AM Labs |
| | | | ❏ Change meds <br> ❏ Call consults <br> ❏ Read consults <br> ❏ Talk with other team members <br> ❏ Test results <br> ❏ Chat with pt and loved ones |
| A/P | | | |

# Index

Page numbers followed by *f* refer to figures; those followed by *t* refer to tables.

# Index

# Index